INTERNATIONAL CASES IN FORENSIC PSYCHOLOGY

This book provides an in-depth investigation of different psychological phenomena in forensic psychology through an analysis of key case studies in the field.

There is a growing requirement for a comprehensive resource that provides practical examples of how forensic psychology models are applied in real-life situations. Filling this lacuna, *International Cases in Forensic Psychology* takes the reader through a series of prominent case studies that illustrate the intricate details of criminal investigations, judicial proceedings, and correctional settings. Drawing on a diverse range of examples from the US, UK, Belgium, Russia, Columbia, Germany, and India which include serial murder, financial deception, and maternal psychosis, Dr. K. Jayasankara Reddy applies psychological theories and methods to understand the intricacies of criminal conduct. These theories range from criminal profiling and behavioral analysis, to the psychology of deceit and the dynamics of influence. Overall, the book will enhance the reader's ability to analyze the fundamental reasons behind criminal behavior and develop more efficient approaches for rehabilitating offenders.

International Cases in Forensic Psychology will be of great interest to students and professionals of forensic psychology, neuropsychology, criminal justice, and related fields.

Dr. K. Jayasankara Reddy is a distinguished expert in neuropsychology, neuroelectrophysiology, and forensic neuropsychology. He earned his M.Sc. and Ph.D. in Psychology specializing in Neuropsychology. Currently, Dr. Reddy is a Professor of Neuropsychology/Cognitive Neuroscience and Dean for Social Sciences at Christ University in Bangalore, India. With a robust academic career spanning teaching, research, and professional practice, he has supervised numerous Ph.D. and M.Phil. candidates, as well as over 100 M.Sc. Psychology research projects.

INTERNATIONAL CASES IN FORENSIC PSYCHOLOGY

Inside the Criminal Mind

K. Jayasankara Reddy

Routledge
Taylor & Francis Group
LONDON AND NEW YORK

Designed cover image: Getty Images / bestdesigns

First published 2025
by Routledge
4 Park Square, Milton Park, Abingdon, Oxon OX14 4RN

and by Routledge
605 Third Avenue, New York, NY 10158

Routledge is an imprint of the Taylor & Francis Group, an informa business

British Library Cataloguing-in-Publication Data
A catalogue record for this book is available from the British Library

ISBN: 978-1-032-98964-8 (hbk)
ISBN: 978-1-032-99206-8 (pbk)
ISBN: 978-1-003-60292-7 (ebk)

DOI: 10.4324/9781003602927

Typeset in Sabon LT Pro
by codeMantra

CONTENTS

ABOUT THE AUTHOR

Dr. K. Jayasankara Reddy is a distinguished scholar and educator renowned for his expertise in the field of forensic neuropsychology. With a career of over two decades, Dr. Reddy has dedicated himself to advancing knowledge and understanding in this complex and vital study area.

Throughout his illustrious career, Dr. Reddy has authored numerous papers and publications, contributing significantly to the academic discourse surrounding forensic neuropsychology. His research has delved into the intricate workings of the human mind, exploring the intersection of psychology and law to shed light on the mysteries of criminal behavior.

In addition to his scholarly endeavors, Dr. Reddy is deeply passionate about education and mentorship. He has served as a dedicated instructor, teaching forensic neuropsychology courses to graduate and undergraduate students. Dr. Reddy's commitment to fostering the next generation of forensic professionals is evident in his tireless efforts to impart knowledge and instill a case-based approach to learning.

Dr. Reddy's mission is to equip forensic students with the knowledge and skills they need to understand the intricacies of the criminal mind. Through his work, he aims to demystify the intricacies of forensic psychology, providing students with a solid foundation rooted in real-world case studies and practical applications.

As the author of *International Cases in Forensic Psychology*, Dr. Reddy brings his wealth of knowledge and experience to bear, offering readers a comprehensive exploration of the fascinating world of investigative psychology. With a keen eye for detail and a passion for unraveling the secrets of famous case studies, Dr. Reddy invites readers on a captivating journey into the depths of the criminal psyche.

PREFACE

Greetings and welcome to *International Cases in Forensic Psychology: Inside the Criminal Mind*. Join me in exploring the connection between psychology and justice as we delve into the depths of the human psyche. The mysterious factors that drive people to engage in criminal behavior have fascinated mankind throughout history. The workings of the criminal psyche, from infamous serial murderers to high-level financial deception, have captivated and confounded experts, law enforcement, and the public.

This book explores investigative psychology, which aims to understand criminal conduct using psychological theories and methods. We explore mysteries within notorious criminal cases throughout history using extensive research, case studies, and real-world examples. Why study the psychology of criminals? What can we learn by understanding the motivations, cognitive processes, and actions of those involved in criminal behavior? These questions guide our pursuit of knowledge in forensic psychology.

The objective of this book is to offer a thorough examination of investigative psychology, spanning various theories, approaches, and applications. We delve into criminal conduct, from profiling and behavioral analysis to the psychology of deceit and influence. Our exploration includes tools and tactics to comprehend and counteract criminal activities. A case-centered methodology connects theoretical principles with real instances. In this book, you will find well-known case studies providing insights into the complexities of criminal conduct and its origins.

This book is more than a compilation of case stories; it is a call to action. By understanding the psychological foundations of criminal conduct, we enhance our ability to address crime's root causes and develop more effective prevention, intervention, and rehabilitation strategies. While reading *International Cases in Forensic Psychology*, approach each case study with an unbiased and analytical mindset. Examine the underlying reasons, recurring behaviors, and psychological interactions involved, and reflect on how these relate to your comprehension of human actions and the need for fairness.

In essence, this book demonstrates how investigative psychology uncovers the hidden aspects of the human mind. By exploring the psyche of wrong-doers, we gain invaluable insights into human behavior and the influences shaping our choices.

PART I

Foundations of Forensic Psychology

1

INTRODUCTION TO FORENSIC PSYCHOLOGY

Introduction

Forensic psychology is a specialized branch that intersects with the legal and criminal justice systems. It involves the application of psychological principles, theories, and methods to understand and address issues related to law and criminal behavior. Forensic psychologists work in various settings, including courts, law enforcement agencies, prisons, and academic institutions, performing assessment, consultation, and research tasks.

One of the primary roles of forensic psychologists is to conduct psychological evaluations for legal purposes. These evaluations can include an assessment of stand trial competency, criminal responsibility (insanity defense), risk of future violence, and sentencing recommendations (Melton et al., 1998). In these contexts, forensic psychologists provide expert testimony to help judges and juries make informed decisions based on psychological findings.

Forensic psychology also involves the study of criminal behavior and the factors that contribute to it. This includes examining the psychological, social, and environmental influences that lead individuals to engage in criminal activities. For example, research has shown that early exposure to violence, substance abuse, and dysfunctional family environments are significant risk factors for criminal behavior (Bartol & Bartol, 2018). By understanding these factors, forensic psychologists can develop interventions and prevention strategies to reduce criminal behavior and recidivism.

Another important aspect of forensic psychology is criminal profiling, which involves analyzing crime scenes and offender behavior to develop profiles of potential suspects. This process, also known as offender profiling, relies on identifying patterns and psychological characteristics consistent with

DOI: 10.4324/9781003602927-2

certain types of crimes (Turvey, 2011). Criminal profilers use this information to assist law enforcement in narrowing down suspect lists and understanding the motivations behind criminal acts.

Forensic psychologists also play a critical role in assessing and treating offenders. This includes working with individuals who have been convicted of crimes to address underlying psychological issues that may contribute to their behavior. Treatment programs often focus on cognitive-behavioral interventions, anger management, substance abuse treatment, and social skills training (Helfgott, 2008). These programs aim to rehabilitate offenders and reduce the likelihood of future criminal behavior.

In addition to working with offenders, forensic psychologists are involved in victim advocacy and support. They provide counseling and support services to victims of crime, helping them cope with the psychological impact of their experiences. This can include trauma-focused therapy, crisis intervention, and legal system assistance (Davies & Beech, 2012). Research is another critical component of forensic psychology. Forensic psychologists conduct studies to understand better various aspects of criminal behavior, legal processes, and the effectiveness of interventions. This research informs evidence-based practices and contributes to the development of policies and procedures within the criminal justice system (Huss, 2013).

Forensic psychology is constantly evolving, with new research and technological advancements shaping its practices. For example, the use of neuroimaging techniques, such as functional magnetic resonance imaging (fMRI), has provided insights into the brain activity of individuals with antisocial personality disorder and other conditions related to criminal behavior (Glenn & Raine, 2014). These advancements could improve forensic psychology assessment and treatment approaches.

In conclusion, forensic psychology is a dynamic and multifaceted field that plays a crucial role in the intersection of psychology and the legal system. Forensic psychologists contribute to understanding and managing criminal behavior through assessment, treatment, research, and consultation. Their work helps to ensure that legal decisions are informed by psychological expertise, ultimately contributing to the fair and effective functioning of the criminal justice system.

References

Bartol, C. R., & Bartol, A. M. (2018). *Introduction to forensic psychology: Research and application*. Sage Publications.

Davies, G. M., & Beech, A. R. (Eds.). (2012). *Forensic psychology: Crime, justice, law, interventions*. John Wiley & Sons.

Glenn, A. L., & Raine, A. (2014). Neurocriminology: Implications for the punishment, prediction, and prevention of criminal behavior. *Nature Reviews Neuroscience*, *15*(1), 54–63.
Helfgott, J. B. (2008). *Criminal behavior: Theories, typologies, and criminal justice*. Sage.
Huss, M. T. (2013). *Forensic psychology: Research, clinical practice, and applications*. John Wiley & Sons.
Melton, G. B., Petrila, J., Poythress, N. G., Slobogin, C., Otto, R. K., & Mossman, D. O. U. G. L. A. S. (1998). Psychological evaluations for the courts: A handbook for mental health professionals and lawyers. *Contemporary Psychology*, *43*, 563–564.
Turvey, B. E. (2011). *Criminal profiling: An introduction to behavioral evidence analysis*. Academic Press.

PART II

Serial Killers and Psychological Profiling

2

CASE STUDY ON TED BUNDY

Introduction

Theodore Robert Bundy, also known as Ted Bundy, was one of the most notorious and prolific American serial killers who killed over 30 women after brutally raping them. He was also described as a necrophile who would occasionally visit the sites at which he had buried his victims and engage in sexual intercourse with their corpses. He was active across seven states, which included Colorado, Utah, Florida, Washington, California, Idaho, and Oregon, between the years 1974 and 1978 and was tried for homicides of young women to which he confessed before being executed in the year 1989. Although he was executed for committing 30 heinous murders, it is estimated that Bundy had killed over 100 women from different age groups, his youngest and last victim being a 12-year-old girl. Bundy, apart from being famous for evading the American police for several years, was also known for having a prominent and normal social, occupational, and personal life, as opposed to what would be expected of a cold-blooded murderer who was on the run for the latter half of his life (Rule, 2012).

Ted Bundy, one of the most infamous serial killers in American history, remains a perplexing and intriguing figure in forensic psychology. His charm, intelligence, and outwardly normal appearance masked a deeply disturbed individual responsible for the brutal murders of numerous women. This case study delves into the psychological profile of Ted Bundy, exploring his background, criminal behavior, and the psychological factors that may have contributed to his actions.

DOI: 10.4324/9781003602927-4

Background

One of the most important biological factors that contribute to crime but remains underrated during conceptualization is gender. Ted Bundy was a male, a gender that is statistically associated with higher crime rates. A study by the Department of Justice in the US reported that between 1980 and 2008, nearly 90% of the offenders were male. Kanazawa and Still (2000) suggested a 20-year window period between the ages of 15 and 34 years when men are most likely to commit gruesome crimes like rape, homicides, and assault. According to sources, Ted Bundy was 28 years old during the onset of his murderous spree, showing that he was within the suggested age group at risk for crime.

Ted Bundy was born to Eleanor Louise Cowell and an unknown father, while his birth certificate mentions an Air Force retired soldier. Louise also mentioned that she was with another war veteran who was the father of Bundy, thus making it very difficult to identify the biological father (Rule, 2012). Some personality traits are genetically inherited, aggression being one among them (Anholt & Mackay, 2012), and a study suggested that about 50% of the variance in aggressive behavior can be explained by genetics (Niv, Tuvblad, Raine, & Baker, 2013). Assuming that he was the child of supposed military veterans, it is possible that Bundy inherited certain traits of aggression and apathy that these veterans possessed as a part of their job. Further, Ted Bundy's maternal grandfather, Sam Cowell, was often described as being a violent man, some taking the claim further that Bundy was the product of Bundy's mother being sexually abused by her own father (Rule, 2012). This could further provide concrete evidence that Bundy was most likely genetically susceptible to aggression. Past psychiatric history within the family showed a history of depression and agoraphobia from the maternal family (Rule, 2012).

Instances like wetting his pants as a sign of protest, having a keen interest in knives, and having a keen interest in death as a child can be suggestive of a difficult temperament, which presents itself as an early disposition to antisocial aggression (Fowles & Dindo, 2009). Bundy was also known to take delight in abusing small animals and bullying younger children as an adolescent. It was also asserted that Ted Bundy's ability to live a dual life was because of his ability to split and compartmentalize different aspects of his life (Rule, 2012). The author of Conversations with a Killer—The Ted Bundy Tapes pointed out that his mother possessed a similar attribute, which had been evident when she heard the tapes in which her son confessed to his crimes and then got up asking the journalist who brought the recording if he wanted desserts.

Ted Bundy was brought up in a family that appeared to belong to a lower socio-economic class, although much information is not available regarding the same. Many studies back the idea that poverty is linked to violent crimes, and Ted Bundy's case might be no different. His family setup was anything but conventional, with instances ranging from being brought up as his own mother's brother to being unaware of his absent, unknown biological father (Rule, 2012). Michaud and Aynesworth (1999, 2019) reported that Bundy's grandfather held extremist views against different races and was known to be abusive. After his mother's marriage to Johnny Bundy, he continued to live in a working-class home in Seattle, away from his familiar surroundings in Philadelphia. The family did not seem to be extremely well off because it is said that his step-father could not indulge his materialistic wishes of lavish things. His mother had four more children after Ted, and, eventually, it can be inferred that he felt neglected (Rule, 2012).

Bundy, further, was described as having a small frame as a teenager and hence socially awkward, making him a subject of bullying in school, which could have led to feelings of shame and embarrassment. This indicated that his peer relationships were poor for the most part of his childhood until he joined college to emerge as a completely different individual. He still had feelings of inferiority associated with class differences between his peers and himself. These negative feelings intensified after knowing the background behind his birth, and multiple accounts stated that he was extremely bitter about his illegitimacy, which affected his relationship with his mother. He also reportedly had early exposure to pornography that contained graphic content, and it was likely that he got it from his grandfather. He also had an affinity for detective novels, true crime documentaries, and magazines that had descriptions of sexual crimes and violence, which indicate that his interest in crimes began early on in life. He further blamed the accessibility and availability of violent images and ideas in the media and said that they primed him to act out violently (Rule, 2012). A study by Huesmann and Taylor (2006) further suggests that fictional violence contributed to both long-term and short-term aggressive behavior, thereby indicating that it could have played a role in his behavior. Given his family circumstances, there seemed to be no supervision that could ensure the censorship of the content that a young Bundy watched. His interview with Michaud suggests that he also abused alcohol before attacking his victims to numb the impulsive feelings to attack first. While already discussed in the psychological effects, it appears that Bundy enjoyed being the person everybody in society knew and feared, giving him a feeling of omnipresence, even after his death.

There has been a lot of interest in Bundy's case, especially from a psychologist's perspective, which views him as a criminal who managed to live a relatively normal life outside his menacing, dark side. As per the timeline, Bundy started his quest for women to kill around the time he had completed his college degree in psychology and joined law school. He was a seemingly bright student and, during his rampage, was also involved in social and political matters, which earned him a recommendation letter from the Republican governor of Washington for his assistance in his campaign. He had a long-term heterosexual relationship that lasted 6 years with Elizabeth Kloepfer, who even said that Bundy helped her through her alcoholism and described him as "warm and kind." He was also working in a suicide hotline crisis center along with working at the Washington State Department Emergency Services, where, despite having an unstable relationship with Carole Ann Boone, she later became his wife after conviction. From his educational and personal history in his early adulthood, there is an obvious sense of stability and security, which is what made him a less likely suspect for the initial tenure of his crimes (Rule, 2012).

Criminal Behavior

Ted Bundy's killing spree began in the mid-1970s and spanned multiple states, including Washington, Oregon, Colorado, Utah, and Florida. He employed a variety of methods to lure his victims, often pretending to be injured or impersonating authority figures to gain their trust. His charm and good looks made it easier for him to attract and deceive young women (Sullivan, 2020).

Bundy's modus operandi involved bludgeoning his victims, followed by sexual assault and sometimes post-mortem mutilation. His behavior exhibited characteristics of organized serial killers, such as meticulous planning, targeting specific victim types, and evading capture for an extended period. He also kept the jewelry of his victims as trophies and even gave some to his female coworkers as gifts. He revisited the sites of disposal of the remains of his victims and engaged in grooming and necrophilia (Keppel & Birnes, 2005).

His first confirmed victim was a student at the University of Washington, Karen Sparks, whom he physically and sexually assaulted brutally such that she incurred permanent brain damage. His first confirmed murder was that of Lynda Ann Haley, who was abducted from her bedroom and sexually assaulted and murdered. His victims shared similar physical characteristics, such as long hair and being a brunette. However, Bundy, in his death row interviews, later denied that he had any specific victim preferences. He went on to commit murders till 1975 when he was caught and imprisoned. In 1977, he escaped out of a courtroom window while appearing for trial, after which he moved to Florida and continued to commit murders till his capture in 1978 (Keppel & Birnes, 2005).

Psychological Profile

Several psychological theories have been proposed to explain Bundy's behavior. One of the most prominent is the concept of psychopathy. Psychopathy is perhaps the most dominant explanation for Bundy's behavior. Defined by a combination of emotional detachment and antisocial tendencies, psychopaths are characterized by their lack of empathy, remorse, or guilt for their actions, as well as their superficial charm and manipulativeness (Hare, 1999). Bundy exemplified these traits in multiple ways. Lack of empathy is one of them. Bundy showed no empathy or remorse for his victims. Despite his charm and intelligence, he was emotionally disconnected from the suffering he caused, viewing his victims more as objects to fulfill his violent desires rather than as human beings.

Bundy's ability to blend into society, appear personable, and lead a double life as a law student and political campaign worker highlights his skill at manipulation. He often lured his victims by pretending to be injured or needing help, exploiting their kindness (Keppel & Birnes, 2005). Bundy was known for his charisma and physical attractiveness, traits he used to his advantage. Many people who met him could not reconcile his charming demeanor with the heinous acts he committed. His ability to gain trust quickly was a hallmark of his psychopathic nature. Psychopathy's focus on shallow emotional affect and a lack of fear or anxiety also explains why Bundy was so confident and calm, even in high-pressure situations like courtroom trials or his multiple escapes from prison. He thrived on the chaos and drama, often seeing it as a game to manipulate those around him.

Bundy's actions also reflected elements of narcissistic personality disorder. His need for admiration, sense of entitlement, and lack of empathy for his victims align with the diagnostic criteria for this disorder (Millon, Simonsen, Birket-Smith, & Davis, 2002). In Bundy's case, he exhibited a belief that he was above others, often boasting about his intelligence, looks, and superiority over those around him. His courtroom behavior, including representing himself and making theatrical statements, reflected his inflated sense of importance. Bundy craved public attention, often basking in the media coverage of his crimes. His dramatic legal defenses, coupled with his desire to prolong his trials, point to his deep-seated need for recognition. The idea of becoming infamous seemed to feed his narcissistic ego. Bundy had no qualms about using people for his own ends, whether it was his romantic partners, victims, or even his own legal team. He viewed others as tools to satisfy his desires or further his image rather than as autonomous individuals. In addition to his need for control, his ability to maintain multiple relationships while committing unspeakable crimes highlights how Bundy compartmentalized his life, another sign of a narcissistic personality structure where one's public image takes precedence over reality.

Sexual sadism is another critical element of Bundy's psychological profile. Sexual sadists derive pleasure from inflicting pain, suffering, or humiliation on others, and Bundy's murders were sexually motivated with a focus on the domination and degradation of his victims (Hickey, 2002).

Bundy's killing spree often involved intense physical violence, and he confessed to necrophiliac tendencies, further indicating his need to dominate and humiliate his victims even after their deaths. His methods of murder, which involved strangulation, mutilation, and sexual assault, highlight his sadistic tendencies. Bundy viewed his victims as objects to control, often keeping their bodies for extended periods post-mortem. His desire for complete dominance over his victims aligns with sexual sadism, as he sought not just to kill but to assert absolute control over another human being's life and body. His sexual sadism combined with psychopathic traits allowed him to carry out his murders without remorse, while the narcissistic traits fueled his belief that he was untouchable, reinforcing his continued patterns of behavior over the years.

Bundy exhibited significant cognitive distortions that allowed him to justify his actions. Like many psychopaths, he likely believed that his victims "deserved" their fate or that they were less than human, which helped him avoid confronting the reality of his crimes. His own statements post-arrest reflect a dehumanizing attitude toward his victims, often referring to them in abstract terms or distancing himself from the severity of his crimes.

Ted Bundy's cognitive distortions played a crucial role in enabling him to carry out his violent actions while maintaining psychological distance from the reality of his crimes. Cognitive distortions, in general, are irrational or biased ways of thinking that distort perception and reality, often used to justify harmful behaviors or alleviate feelings of guilt. For Bundy, these distortions were vital in his ability to repeatedly murder and assault women while maintaining a sense of internal justification and emotional detachment.

Bundy consistently dehumanized his victims, seeing them as objects rather than individuals with their own lives, emotions, and values. This form of cognitive distortion is often found in individuals with psychopathic tendencies, as it allows them to bypass normal human empathy. By reducing his victims to mere tools for his gratification, Bundy was able to suppress any moral or emotional conflict that might arise from his actions. Post-arrest, Bundy often referred to his victims in clinical or abstract terms, which further reinforced the emotional distance he maintained. Instead of acknowledging the humanity of the women he killed, he spoke of them in detached terms, treating his violent acts as though they were experiments or expressions of power rather than atrocities against real people. This linguistic detachment was a key part of his cognitive strategy to avoid guilt or moral reckoning.

Another distortion that Bundy likely employed was the minimization of the harm he inflicted. By downplaying the suffering he caused, he could avoid fully confronting the magnitude of his actions. For instance, he may have convinced himself that his victims did not suffer much or that their lives were less important compared to his own desires. In his worldview, the needs of others were secondary, and this allowed him to rationalize his behavior as fulfilling his own sense of entitlement. He likely justified that his violent acts were part of his "right" or that his personal needs (whether sexual, emotional, or related to control) took precedence over the basic human rights of his victims. Bundy often externalized the blame for his actions.

He hinted in interviews that his behavior was influenced by external factors, such as pornography, suggesting that his actions were not entirely under his control. This externalization of blame is a common cognitive distortion in offenders, allowing them to avoid full accountability for their crimes. By placing blame on external forces, Bundy could mitigate his sense of personal responsibility. He portrayed himself as a victim of circumstance or societal influences, which served as a mental buffer against fully recognizing the intrinsic nature of his violence. This type of cognitive distortion allowed him to believe that he was not inherently evil but instead a product of environmental triggers, thus lessening the moral weight of his actions.

Bundy's cognitive distortions did more than just allow him to avoid guilt—they actively fueled his ability to maintain a double life. His distorted thinking patterns helped him compartmentalize his existence: on one side, he was a charming, intelligent man involved in law and politics, while, on the other, he was a brutal serial killer. The cognitive dissonance that most people would experience in this situation was avoided through these distortions, enabling him to appear outwardly normal while continuing his crimes.

Bundy's statements after his arrest further exemplify how deeply ingrained these cognitive distortions were in his psychology. When speaking about his crimes, he rarely showed empathy or expressed genuine remorse. Instead, he spoke with a cold detachment, often focusing on himself rather than his victims. This further illustrates his profound disconnection from the humanity of those he killed, a hallmark of both his psychopathic tendencies and his reliance on cognitive distortions to maintain his self-image.

Possible Treatment

Given the complexity of Ted Bundy's psychological profile, treatment would have been extraordinarily challenging. Psychopathy, narcissistic personality disorder, and sexual sadism are notoriously resistant to treatment. Traditional therapeutic approaches, such as cognitive-behavioral therapy (CBT), might have offered limited benefits. CBT could potentially help in addressing some of the cognitive distortions and maladaptive thought patterns, but its effectiveness with individuals exhibiting psychopathic traits is limited due to their inherent lack of empathy and manipulative tendencies (Hare, 1999).

Medication could also be considered as part of a treatment plan, particularly for managing impulsive behaviors and co-occurring conditions like depression or anxiety. However, there is no medication specifically approved for treating psychopathy or narcissistic personality disorder (Hickey, 2002).

Some research suggests that early intervention and consistent, long-term therapeutic engagement might help manage certain behaviors. Programs focusing on enhancing social skills, increasing prosocial behavior, and developing empathy might be beneficial, although their success in highly psychopathic individuals is questionable (Millon et al., 2002).

In Bundy's case, the lack of early intervention and the severity of his disorders likely rendered most conventional treatments ineffective. His high level of intelligence and manipulative skills would also pose significant challenges in a therapeutic setting, as he could easily deceive and manipulate therapists (Keppel & Birnes, 2005).

Captivity and Trial

Bundy's ability to evade capture for so long can be attributed to his intelligence and cunning. He often altered his appearance and used different aliases to avoid detection. However, his arrogance eventually led to his downfall. In 1978, Bundy was arrested in Florida after a series of careless mistakes, including driving a stolen vehicle (Rule, 2012).

During his trial, Bundy chose to represent himself, displaying his confidence and belief in his own abilities. His courtroom demeanor further highlighted his manipulative and narcissistic traits. Despite his efforts, Bundy was convicted of multiple murders and sentenced to death (Michaud & Aynesworth, 2012).

Conclusion

Ted Bundy's case continues to be a subject of fascination and study in forensic psychology. His ability to blend into society, coupled with his horrific crimes, provides a chilling example of how dangerous individuals can hide in plain sight. Understanding Bundy's psychological makeup offers valuable insights into the minds of serial killers and underscores the importance of early intervention and treatment for individuals displaying psychopathic tendencies.

References

Anholt, R. R., & Mackay, T. F. (2012). Genetics of aggression. *Annual Review of Genetics*, *46*, 145–164.

Fowles, D. C., & Dindo, L. (2009). Temperament and psychopathy: A dual-pathway model. *Current Directions in Psychological Science*, *18*(3), 179–183.

Hare, R. D. (1999). *Without conscience: The disturbing world of the psychopaths among us*. Guilford Press.

Hickey, E. W. (2002). *Serial murderers and their victims* (p. 448). Wadsworth Pub.

Huesmann, L. R., & Taylor, L. D. (2006). The role of media violence in violent behavior. *Annual Review of Public Health*, *27*, 393–415.

Kanazawa, S., & Still, M. C. (2000). Why men commit crimes (and why they desist). *Sociological Theory*, *18*(3), 434–447.
Keppel, R. D., & Birnes, W. J. (2005). *The riverman: Ted Bundy and I hunt for the green river killer*. Pocket Books.
Michaud, S. G., & Aynesworth, H. (1999). *The only living witness: The true story of serial sex killer Ted Bundy*. Authorlink.
Michaud, S. G., & Aynesworth, H. (2000). *Ted Bundy: Conversations with a killer: The death row interviews*. Union Square & Co.
Millon, T., Simonsen, E., Birket-Smith, M., & Davis, R. D. (Eds.). (2002). *Psychopathy: Antisocial, criminal, and violent behavior*. The Guilford Press.
Niv, S., Tuvblad, C., Raine, A., & Baker, L. A. (2013). Aggression and rule-breaking: Heritability and stability of antisocial behavior problems in childhood and adolescence. *Journal of Criminal Justice*, *41*(5), 285–291.
Rule, A. (2012). *The stranger beside me*. Planet Ann Rule.
Sullivan, K. M. (2020). *The Bundy murders: A comprehensive history*. McFarland.

3

CASE STUDY ON JEFFREY DAHMER

Introduction

Jeffery Lionel Dahmer was a convicted American serial killer, a sex offender, a cannibal, and someone who engaged in necrophilia. He had committed a total of 17 murders between the year of 1978 and 1991. He was born on May 21, 1960, in Milwaukee, Wisconsin, US. He died on November 28, 1994. He was killed by one of his fellow prison inmates in jail (Fido, 1995).

Jeffrey Dahmer, also known as the Milwaukee Cannibal, committed some of the most gruesome and disturbing crimes in modern history. His case continues to be studied extensively within forensic psychology due to the shocking nature of his actions and the complex psychological profile he presents. This case study explores Dahmer's background, criminal behavior, psychological profile, potential treatments, and the details of his captivation and trial.

Jeffrey Dahmer's reign of terror spanned over a decade, during which he lured young men to his apartment, where he would kill, dismember, and often engage in acts of necrophilia and cannibalism (Fido, 1995). Understanding Dahmer's mind provides valuable insights into the psychological and environmental factors that can contribute to such extreme criminal behavior.

Background

Jeffrey Dahmer was born on May 21, 1960, in Milwaukee, Wisconsin. His early life was marked by instability and isolation. Dahmer exhibited signs of abandonment and neglect, particularly after his parents' turbulent relationship led to their divorce. He developed an early fascination with dead

DOI: 10.4324/9781003602927-5

animals, which he would collect and dissect, hinting at his later morbid interests (Schwartz, 1992).

Dahmer struggled with alcoholism from a young age, which exacerbated his social isolation and contributed to his inability to form meaningful relationships. Despite these early warning signs, Dahmer managed to graduate from high school and briefly attended Ohio State University before dropping out due to his drinking problem (Davis, 1991).

When we look at the biological perspective, we observe that Jeffery Dahmer could have been biologically predisposed to mental health concerns. In a brief glimpse into his past, we observe that his mother, Joyce Dahmer, was often depressed and sought attention from her husband, who was busy obtaining a degree from the university and, in turn, neglecting his wife and children. To seek her husband's attention, Joyce Dahmer got addicted to Equanil pills and also attempted suicide. Since we know that Jeffery Dahmer was addicted to alcohol, it is safe for us to deduce that addiction runs in his family since his mother got easily addicted to drugs as well (Fido, 1995). According to a study by Li (2000), individuals can be predisposed to alcoholism, which could also result in impulsivity and novelty seeking.

As a child, Jeffery Dahmer suffered from a double hernia, which could have made him constitutionally weak, which could have had an effect on him psychologically as well. As a child, he was considered very weak and often stayed in his room. Hence, the hernia surgery could have left him physiologically weak as a child (Fido, 1995). When we come to know about Jeffery Dahmer's alcohol addiction, we discover it was probably an escape route from the reality around him. But alcohol brings about chemical changes in the body, from disinhibiting behavior to making a person act more erratic and impulsive, to withdrawal symptoms, and an urge to drink more. And repeat the cycle all over again. As we say that everything that is psychological is biological; if we look at Dahmer's behavior, we observe that he felt no empathy or a sense of remorse when he murdering his victims. Instead, he was sexually aroused when he looked at corpses, and it excited him. The emotional center of the brain is the limbic system, which consists of the amygdala, which is the seat of emotions in the brain. We can assume that there could have been structural as well as functional dysfunction that could have caused emotional blunting specifically related to fear and remorse. A study by Stone, Cosmides, Tooby, Kroll and Knight (2002) found that social exchange among individuals who have a deficit in the limbic system can be selectively impaired and they lack an overall social intelligence quotient.

Now, we come to Jeffery Dahmer's social perspective. He learned a lot from his father when it came to preserving corpses and preserving the bones of animals. He was even encouraged by his father. Jeffery Dahmer was a social isolate, so whenever he engaged in something, his father encouraged it—when Jeffery showed interest in his father's activities, his father felt as if his son wished to connect with him, but, unfortunately, his son had other motives. When we discuss Jeffery Dahmer's school life, we come across the fact that he was not much of a social child. He liked to be alone. His friends considered him "weird" and a "freak" because he collected carcasses of insects and stored them in jars. In his later childhood and early adolescence, he started to play pranks on his classmates, and he later became the class clown. He became a source of amusement. This behavior of Dahmer possibly indicated that he wanted to be socially accepted and didn't want his social identity to be that of a loner. He used to perform mimicry, even though it was morbid to be liked and approved socially by others. Another out-of-the-ordinary thing that happened was that Jeffery Dahmer started to drink alcohol in class at the age of 14 years. This disturbed his other classmates as well, but for him it was a ""coping mechanism" that no doubt was maladaptive. This could have led to disinhibited behavior, which he could havc coped with in social settings, but Jeffery did not have a strong support system either. He didn't have a friend group, and his family was dysfunctional as well. His parents sought counseling, but it was unsuccessful, and this led to a divorce. Jeffery Dahmer's parents started to fight in front of the children, and later Dahmer had to move to his grandmother's house because it became too uncomfortable and unbearable for him to live in that house. Dahmer joined the army, where he was always stressed and often got into fights with his colleagues. It was even reported that Dahmer had raped two of the soldiers. Since Dahmer was always socially cut off from his friends, his peers, and also his family, he started to look at everyone as an object. He didn't attach emotions to anyone. He always attempted to find gratification and satisfaction from people without considering them as humans (Fido, 1995). A study by Viding and McCrory (2019) focused on the fact that psychopaths tend to have a reduced motivation to develop relationships that are authentic in nature.

Dahmer had experiences that validated his distorted thoughts. One of these incidents was when Dahmer was offered money to allow another man to engage in sexual activities with him. He was once arrested for masturbating in front of two 12-year-old boys in a park. He began to think in the same pattern and then started to find his victim in gay bathhouses and pubs, where he would carefully select his victims (Fido, 1995). A study of successful psychopaths indicates that their behavior is annotated by boldness, disinhibited behavior, conscientiousness, and fearless dominance (Lilienfeld, Watts, & Smith, 2015). Jeffery Dahmer might have lacked social skills, but he knew very well how to manipulate people and use them for his own benefit.

Criminal Behavior

Dahmer's killing spree began in 1978 when he murdered his first victim, a hitchhiker named Steven Hicks. After a 9-year hiatus, during which he attempted to suppress his urges, Dahmer resumed his killings in 1987. Over the next few years, he murdered 16 more young men, employing methods such as drugging, strangling, and dismembering his victims (Silva, Ferrari & Leong, 2002).

Dahmer's first murder happened after graduating secondary school, in June 1978, when he got a drifter named Steven Hicks and took him home. Dahmer slaughtered him by striking him in the head and choking him with a free weight. Dahmer dissected the corpse of his first victim, stuffed the body parts in plastic bags, and hid them behind his folks' home. He later uncovered the remaining parts, broke the bones with a heavy hammer, and dissipated them in a faraway place. It wasn't until September 1987 that Dahmer took his second victim, Steven Tuomi. Dahmer lured Tuomi to a hotel and rented a room, and Dahmer, in the end, woke up to discover Tuomi dead, with no memory of the previous night. He purchased a huge bag to move the body to his grandmother's cellar, where he dissected and masturbated on the body before discarding the remaining parts. At his grandmother's home, Dahmer executed another two victims, but by this time, his grandmother was tired of Dahmer's alcoholism and late-night rendezvous and removed him from her premises; she was, however, oblivious about his heinous acts (Fido, 1995).

In September 1989, he was convicted of child sexual abuse and assault. While waiting for his sentence, he went back to his grandmother's place and sodomized, took pictures, strangled, dismembered, and drugged Anthony Sears, an aspiring model. Over the accompanying 2 years, Dahmer's victim tally quickened, carrying his aggregate from 4 to 17. As he advanced, he started to explore different avenues regarding chemical methods to dispose of the bodies after consuming them. Dahmer likewise administered unrefined lobotomies, penetrating into victims' skulls with muriatic acid while keeping them alive. On May 27, 1991, Dahmer's neighbor Sandra Smith called the police to report that an Asian kid was running away in the road. When the police arrived, the boy was too shocked to speak, and Dahmer told the police that the boy was his 19-year-old boyfriend. In reality, the boy was 14 years old, and he was the younger brother of the Laotian boy whom Dahmer had molested previously (Fido, 1995).

The police accompanied Dahmer and the youngster home. Not wanting to get entangled in problems of homosexual relationships, they took just a careless glance around before leaving. When the police left the scene, Dahmer murdered the teen and continued with his usual customs. Had the police led even a fundamental hunt, they would have discovered the body of Tony Hughes, Dahmer's 12th victim. Prior to being arrested, Jeffery Dahmer had murdered four more men. Two police officers were taken straight to Dahmer's house when they found a young man named Tracy Edward with handcuffs on, walking by the road, reporting that he was drugged and restrained by a "weird man." Further investigation led to body parts frozen in the refrigerator and a collection of grotesque pictures of his victims. Dahmer was found guilty of all of the crimes that he had committed despite his pleading "not guilty" and "plea for insanity." He was sentenced to life imprisonment, but he was later killed by an inmate named Christopher Scarver (Fido, 1995).

Dahmer's criminal behavior was characterized by a ritualistic pattern. He often lured victims to his apartment with promises of money or alcohol, incapacitated them with drugs, and then proceeded to kill them. Dahmer would engage in acts of necrophilia and cannibalism, preserving body parts as macabre trophies (Ressler & Shachtman, 1997).

Psychological Profile

Jeffrey Dahmer, one of the most notorious serial killers in modern history, presents a psychological profile that is both multifaceted and disturbing. His actions—spanning from 1978 to his arrest in 1991—resulted in the deaths of 17 young men. Beyond the murders, Dahmer's crimes included necrophilia, cannibalism, and attempts to create zombified victims through crude lobotomies (Fido, 1995). Understanding the psychological underpinnings of such extreme behavior requires an examination of various personality disorders, paraphilias, and cognitive distortions that coalesced to form Dahmer's pathology.

Dahmer exhibited many signs of borderline personality disorder (BPD), which is characterized by instability in interpersonal relationships, poor self-image, and emotional regulation. A common feature of BPD is a deep fear of abandonment, and this fear appears to have been a significant driving force behind Dahmer's actions. From an early age, Dahmer exhibited signs of social isolation, and his parents' tumultuous relationship further exacerbated his emotional instability. This fear of abandonment—especially after his parents' divorce—manifested in his obsessive need to control and possess others. In his relationships, Dahmer demonstrated classic BPD traits. One of Dahmer's primary motives was his overwhelming fear of being left alone. In interviews, Dahmer himself admitted that he murdered and then performed horrific acts on his victims because he wanted to create submissive, passive partners who would never leave him. His attempts to turn his victims into "zombies" by drilling holes into their skulls and injecting acid were driven by his desperate desire to keep them around indefinitely, rendering them completely submissive and dependent (Fido, 1995). Dahmer's struggle with his sexual identity also likely contributed to his sense of inner turmoil. He lived a closeted life, and his inability to reconcile his sexual orientation with societal norms created a deep sense of shame and self-hatred. This conflict further fueled his need to dominate others and project his fantasies of control onto his victims. Dahmer described his sense of inner emptiness, which is a hallmark of BPD. He sought extreme forms of stimulation—such as necrophilia and cannibalism—as ways to fill this void. His crimes can be viewed as attempts to quell the deep loneliness he felt throughout his life.

In addition to BPD, Dahmer's behavior and thought patterns reflected elements of schizotypal personality disorder (SPD). Individuals with SPD often exhibit eccentric behaviors, unusual thinking, and discomfort in close relationships. Though Dahmer's most obvious traits might align with antisocial personality disorder (ASPD), his peculiar and bizarre thoughts align with the criteria of schizotypal disorder, particularly his distorted sense of reality and detachment from normal societal values. Dahmer's desire to control his victims extended beyond murder into deeply bizarre rituals. He engaged in necrophilia and cannibalism, preserving body parts and creating shrines of his victims' remains (Fido, 1995). These actions point to a distorted sense of reality, where Dahmer attempted to immortalize his victims and create a personal world where he could dominate without consequence. His fascination with body parts and his creation of an altar made from bones and skulls also highlight his unusual thought processes and detachment from conventional human interaction. Dahmer struggled with social relationships from an early age, preferring isolation and avoiding deep connections. His inability to form close bonds with others is a core trait of SPD, as individuals with this condition often experience intense discomfort in social settings and exhibit difficulty forming meaningful relationships. Dahmer's sense of alienation and inability to interact in socially acceptable ways further contributed to his eventual resort to extreme forms of control and violence to maintain relationships on his terms.

At the core of Dahmer's psychological makeup were his paraphilic tendencies, most notably **necrophilia** and **cannibalism**. Paraphilic disorders involve intense, persistent sexual interests in atypical objects, activities, or situations, often leading to harmful consequences for others. In Dahmer's case, these deviant sexual interests were central to his criminal behavior, driving him to commit acts of murder in service of fulfilling his fantasies.

Dahmer's necrophilia—his sexual attraction to dead bodies—was one of the most shocking aspects of his behavior. He killed not only to eliminate resistance from his victims but also to engage in sexual acts with their lifeless bodies. Necrophilia provided Dahmer with complete control over his victims, allowing him to enact his fantasies without any fear of rejection or abandonment. For Dahmer, having sex with his victims' corpses represented the ultimate form of possession, where his partner would never leave or resist him. Cannibalism, another feature of Dahmer's crimes, was linked to his need for control and ownership. Dahmer admitted that consuming parts of his victims made him feel as though they had become a permanent part of him. Eating his victims was a way to assert dominance and symbolically preserve their presence within him forever. Dahmer's desire to possess and consume others speaks to the extreme nature of his paraphilias, as he sought to transcend physical separation by literally ingesting his victims. Dahmer's crimes reveal an overwhelming compulsion to possess, control, and dominate others in ways that bypass normal human boundaries. His paraphilic disorders were not just sexual interests; they were deeply embedded in his need to control his environment and relationships. This obsession with power, taken to the extreme, is what ultimately fueled his crimes.

Dahmer's psychological profile also shows traits of **Antisocial Personality Disorder (ASPD)**, particularly in his disregard for the rights of others, lack of empathy, and repeated unlawful behavior. ASPD is characterized by a pattern of socially irresponsible, exploitative, and guiltless behavior, and Dahmer exhibited many of these traits throughout his life. Dahmer's ability to kill repeatedly without showing any real remorse or guilt is indicative of ASPD. His confessions after his arrest did not come with expressions of regret or moral reflection but, instead, a cold rccounting of events. Dahmer's lack of concern for the suffering of his victims or their families is a hallmark of ASPD, where individuals are unable or unwilling to consider the impact of their actions on others. Dahmer's criminal behavior escalated over time, moving from petty theft and alcohol abuse to increasingly violent and depraved acts. His ability to continue killing, despite the risk of being caught, shows his disregard for social rules and norms. Even when apprehended by law enforcement in certain instances, such as when a young victim escaped and was returned to him by police, Dahmer was able to manipulate the situation, showing his skill in deceiving others and evading capture.

This demonstrates his deep-seated disregard for societal expectations and his sense of entitlement to act outside the boundaries of law and morality. Unlike many individuals with ASPD, Dahmer was able to blend into society for much of his life. While many with ASPD exhibit overtly aggressive or impulsive behavior, Dahmer was more reserved and calculated. His ability to maintain jobs and relationships, as well as his semblance of normalcy, sets him apart from more impulsive or outwardly hostile individuals with ASPD. He did not exhibit the grandiosity or outward arrogance seen in some psychopathic killers, but his calm, detached demeanor allowed him to maintain a dual life for years, avoiding suspicion despite his horrific crimes.

Jeffrey Dahmer's actions were underpinned by a series of cognitive distortions—irrational ways of thinking that allowed him to justify and rationalize his horrific behavior. These distortions helped him maintain his internal sense of control and reduce any cognitive dissonance that might arise from his crimes.

Like other serial killers, Dahmer dehumanized his victims, viewing them not as individuals with their own lives and rights but as objects to be controlled and manipulated. This dehumanization made it easier for Dahmer to commit acts of extreme violence without experiencing guilt. His victims became merely tools for him to act out his fantasies, devoid of any personal identity or humanity in his eyes. Dahmer may have minimized the harm he was causing in his mind, convincing himself that his actions were justified or inevitable. By focusing on his own desires and needs, Dahmer likely downplayed the suffering of his victims, viewing their pain and death as secondary to his pursuit of control and fulfillment. This cognitive distortion allowed him to persist in his behavior without facing the moral weight of his actions. Dahmer also showed tendencies to externalize blame for his actions. In interviews, he suggested that his fascination with death and control was beyond his ability to stop, as though he were driven by forces outside of his control.

Possible Treatment

Treating an individual with Jeffrey Dahmer's psychological profile would be extraordinarily challenging. His combination of paraphilic disorders, personality disorders, and profound, deviant urges would likely resist conventional therapeutic interventions. Cognitive-behavioral therapy (CBT) might address some cognitive distortions and maladaptive thought patterns, but its effectiveness would be limited due to deep-seated and highly specific paraphilic interests. Additionally, psychopathy, as indicated by his lack of empathy and remorse, generally shows poor responsiveness to treatment (Hare, 1999).

Medications might be used to manage associated conditions such as depression or anxiety, but there is no pharmacological treatment for paraphilic disorders or personality disorders. Long-term incarceration and isolation would likely be the most effective way to manage the risk he posed to society (Stone, 2001).

Captivation and Trial

Jeffrey Dahmer was finally apprehended on July 22, 1991, when one of his intended victims, Tracy Edwards, managed to escape and alert the police. Upon entering Dahmer's apartment, authorities discovered a scene of unimaginable horror, including human remains, photographs of dismembered bodies, and a collection of preserved skulls (Davis, 1991).

During his trial, Dahmer pleaded guilty but insane to 15 counts of murder. His defense team argued that his actions were the result of severe mental illness, while the prosecution maintained that he was fully aware of the wrongfulness of his actions. The jury ultimately found Dahmer legally sane, and he was sentenced to 15 consecutive life terms in prison (Silva et al., 2002).

Conclusion

Jeffrey Dahmer's case continues to captivate and horrify, offering profound insights into the darkest corners of the human psyche. His ability to hide his monstrous acts behind a veneer of normalcy challenges our understanding of criminal behavior and the factors that drive individuals to commit such heinous crimes. Studying Dahmer's psychological profile underscores the importance of early intervention and comprehensive mental health care to potentially prevent similar tragedies.

References

Davis, D. A. (1991). *The Jeffrey Dahmer story: An American nightmare*. St. Martin's Paperbacks.

Fido, M. (1995). *Twentieth-century murder: A year-by-year account of the world's most pitiless crimes*.

Hare, R. D. (1999). *Without conscience: The disturbing world of the psychopaths among us*. Guilford Press.

Li, T. K. (2000). Pharmacogenetics of responses to alcohol and genes that influence alcohol drinking. *Journal of Studies on Alcohol*, *61*(1), 5–12. https://doi.org/10.15288/jsa.2000.61.5

Lilienfeld, S. O., Watts, A. L., & Smith, S. F. (2015). Successful psychopathy. *Current Directions in Psychological Science*, *24*(4), 298–303. https://doi.org/10.1177/0963721415580297

Ressler, R. K., & Shachtman, T. (1997). *I have lived in the monster: A report from the Abyss*. St. Martin's Press.

Schwartz, H. (1992). *The alchemy of murder: The mind behind the mask*. University of Chicago Press.

Silva, J. A., Ferrari, M. M., & Leong, G. B. (2002). The case of Jeffrey Dahmer: Sexual serial homicide from a neuropsychiatric developmental perspective. *Journal of Forensic Sciences*, *47*(6), 1347–1359.

Stone, M. H. (2001). Serial killers: An epidemiological study of their mental disorders. *American Journal of Psychiatry*, *158*(6), 903–908.

Stone, V. E., Cosmides, L., Tooby, J., Kroll, N., & Knight, R. T. (2002). Selective impairment of reasoning about social exchange in a patient with bilateral limbic system damage. *Proceedings of the National Academy of Sciences*, *99*(17), 11531–11536. https://doi.org/10.1073/pnas.122352699

Viding, E., & McCrory, E. (2019). Towards understanding atypical social affiliation in psychopathy. *The Lancet Psychiatry*, *6*(5), 437–444. https://doi.org/10.1016/s2215-0366(19)30049-5

4

JACK THE RIPPER

A Psychological Profile

Introduction

The Jack the Ripper murders have secured themselves in the annals of criminal history as the most excellent whodunit murder case in the world. The murders occurred in 1888, when policing techniques were in their infancy and forensic knowledge was practically nonexistent. There was no signed confession and no official arrest, so proof of the Ripper's identity has remained unknown for over 130 years (Evans & Rumbelow, 2006).

Today, the Ripper is regarded as the "father" of the modern-day serial killer. It was the first recorded case of a serial killer in the UK and, at the time, caused a mass hysteria in the public imagination and in the numerous columns of newspapers. The entire city of London was under the Ripper's shadow, and the grim legacy still lingers today around the back streets of Whitechapel (Evans & Rumbelow, 2006). But what kind of man was he? What drove his murderous rampage?

The case of Jack the Ripper is a landmark in criminal history and forensic psychology, marking one of the earliest instances of serial murder to receive widespread media attention. The Ripper's brutal killing spree left a lasting legacy, influencing the fields of criminology, forensic science, and criminal profiling. This case study delves into the enigmatic mind of Jack the Ripper, exploring the psychological and societal factors that may have contributed to his reign of terror.

DOI: 10.4324/9781003602927-6

Background

Jack the Ripper remains one of the most infamous and mysterious serial killers in history. Operating in the Whitechapel district of London in 1888, he committed a series of brutal murders that shocked and terrified the public. Despite numerous investigations and theories, Jack the Ripper's identity has never been definitively established (Evans & Rumbelow, 2006). This case study examines the background, criminal behavior, psychological profile, possible treatment, and the investigation surrounding this notorious figure.

In the late 19th century, London's East End was a densely populated, poverty-stricken area plagued by crime and disease. The socio-economic conditions of Whitechapel created an environment ripe for criminal activity. The victims of Jack the Ripper were primarily women engaged in prostitution, a common means of survival in such dire circumstances (Evans & Rumbelow, 2006).

The Ripper's first known victim, Mary Ann Nichols, was discovered on August 31, 1888. Over the next few months, four more women—Annie Chapman, Elizabeth Stride, Catherine Eddowes, and Mary Jane Kelly—were found murdered and mutilated in a similar fashion. The savagery of the crimes and the Ripper's apparent anatomical knowledge suggested a deeply disturbed individual with a methodical approach to killing (Cook, 2009).

Since the bodies of the victims when they were found were still warm, there were vague eyewitness descriptions of the Ripper, and composite sketches were made. Ripper was described as a man between the ages of 25 and 35, between 5'2 and 5'7 in height, wearing a felt hat and jacket that covered most of his facial features. Considering the physical strength needed to carry out the murder and mutilations, we can also hypothesize that he would have been healthy and strong. At that time, police had many suspects from both the upper and lower strata of society. There was even some speculation that the Freemasons were orchestrating the murders and that the killings were the work of a group of men rather than a single individual (Keppel, Weis, Brown, & Welch, 2005).

Criminal Behavior

Jack the Ripper's modus operandi involved attacking women in secluded areas, often late at night or in the early morning. The victims were typically strangled before having their throats cut and bodies mutilated. The precision of the mutilations, particularly the removal of internal organs, indicated a certain level of anatomical knowledge, leading some to speculate that the Ripper had medical or surgical training (Begg, 2013).

The escalation in brutality with each subsequent murder suggested growing confidence and boldness on the part of the killer. The ferocity and ritualistic nature of the mutilations pointed toward a sadistic personality, possibly driven by deep-seated anger or psychosexual motivations (Rumbelow, 2004).

Forty-three-year-old Mary Ann Nichols, or Polly Nichols, was the first victim who had all the signatures of Ripper. She was found in unfrequented yards in Buck Rows of Whitechapel, lying in a pool of her own blood. There was a deep slash to her throat, cut from left ear to right ear, such that her head was almost separated from the rest of her body. Her clothes were scrunched up to her stomach such that her abdomen was exposed. Her face was bruised, and her teeth were missing, indicating she was beaten severely. Other wounds include a deep slashing around her stomach region, which also caused internal damage, and two stab wounds to her vagina (Keppel et al., 2005).

The next victim, Annie Chapman, was found dead near a stable yard in a similar manner. She had incurred more bruises to her face and torso, with her internal organs missing, including parts of her abdomen, uterus, parts of vagina, and bladder. The killer had objects of her possession laid on display beside her and had forcefully removed the ring from her ring finger. A few days later, Elizabeth Stride, a 45-year-old prostitute, was found with her neck slashed open from left to right, without any reports of other mutilations on her body. On the same evening, the mutilated remains of Catherine Eddowes were found with the throat slashed, the kidney and uterus missing, lips and nose must, and related stab wounds to the liver and groin (Keppel et al., 2005).

The last victim, Mary Jane Kelly, a 24- to 25-year-old prostitute, was the most anomalous of all the victims of Ripper in terms of her age, level of mutilation, and body display. Kelly was killed by a deep cut to her throat, a signature of Ripper killings. Her nose and lips were mutilated, and her face was almost ripped off of her skeleton. Many organs were removed from her remains, and, unlike in the case of other victims, they were found displayed around her body (Keppel et al., 2005).

Many other women whose murders share similarities with the Ripper killings were attributed to be the work of the Ripper. However, none of these murders have been officially recognized as Ripper's victims. Another key aspect of the Ripper case was the letters received by a London news agency, allegedly written and signed by Jack the Ripper, taunting the police. There are varying opinions by experts as to whether letters were actually written by the killer or if it was written by someone trying to mislead the police (Keppel et al., 2005).

Psychological Profile

Creating a psychological profile of Jack the Ripper involves examining the patterns and characteristics of his crimes. Modern criminal profiling techniques suggest that the Ripper may have been a white male in his late twenties to early thirties, living locally in Whitechapel. His intimate knowledge of the area and ability to evade capture indicate a familiarity with the district and its inhabitants (Douglas & Olshaker, 1997).

Jack the Ripper is one of the most infamous and enigmatic figures in criminal history. Operating in London's Whitechapel district during the fall of 1888, this unknown serial killer is believed to have brutally murdered at least five women, all of whom were prostitutes. The sheer savagery of the killings, combined with the Ripper's ability to evade capture, has turned him into an enduring mystery (Douglas & Olshaker, 1997). While no definitive identity has ever been established, criminologists and psychologists have analyzed the Ripper's actions in order to construct a psychological profile of the man behind the murders. This profile is based on the behaviors displayed at the crime scenes, the known victimology, and historical context and incorporates elements of forensic psychology, personality theory, and criminal profiling. The murders attributed to Jack the Ripper were distinguished by a combination of precision and extreme brutality. In each case, the Ripper not only killed his victims but mutilated their bodies, often removing organs in what appeared to be a deliberate and methodical manner. This combination of cold, calculated behavior and intense violence suggests that Jack the Ripper exhibited traits of psychopathy.

Psychopathy is a personality disorder characterized by a lack of empathy, superficial charm, grandiosity, and impulsive behavior, often accompanied by criminal or violent tendencies. Though the term was not used in the 19th century, the profile of Jack the Ripper matches modern conceptions of psychopathy, especially regarding his lack of empathy for his victims and his ability to commit atrocities without displaying any outward signs of emotional distress (Hare, 1999).

The Ripper's ability to stalk, kill, and mutilate his victims without showing remorse or concern for the humanity of his victims points to a deep level of callousness. Psychopaths are known for their emotional detachment and their tendency to view people as objects rather than human beings. This detachment allows them to commit violent acts without feeling guilt or remorse. In the case of Jack the Ripper, this callousness is evidenced by the way he treated his victims, reducing them to mere objects of violence and degradation.

The mutilation of the Ripper's victims suggests a psychological need for control and domination. The fact that he often removed specific organs, such as the uterus or kidneys, demonstrates a fixation on exerting power over the bodies of his victims, beyond mere killing. This level of post-mortem mutilation indicates that Jack the Ripper likely derived a sense of empowerment from his crimes, seeing himself as a master over life and death. Many psychopaths exhibit a sense of grandiosity, where they feel superior to others and seek to assert their control. The Ripper's choice of victims—vulnerable, impoverished women—further underscores his need for dominance over those he perceived as weak or powerless.

Despite the horrific nature of his crimes, Jack the Ripper was able to blend into the working-class environment of Whitechapel. Like many psychopaths, the Ripper may have appeared normal or even charming, allowing him to gain the trust of his victims and lure them into secluded areas where he could strike. His ability to move unnoticed and escape after committing such brutal murders suggests that he was capable of concealing his true nature, much like many modern-day psychopaths who can maintain outward appearances while harboring violent tendencies.

One of the more prominent theories about Jack the Ripper is that he was driven by **sexual sadism**—a paraphilia in which an individual derives sexual gratification from inflicting pain, suffering, or humiliation on others. While it is unclear whether the Ripper sexually assaulted his victims in a conventional sense, the sheer brutality of his attacks and the focus on female reproductive organs suggests that his motivations were at least partially sexual. In several of the Ripper murders, the killer targeted the genital area of his victims, often mutilating their bodies in ways that suggest sexual symbolism. This form of mutilation, which appears to have had no practical purpose, indicates that Jack the Ripper may have derived a sense of pleasure from the symbolic violation of his victims. This aligns with patterns seen in sexual sadists, who often engage in acts of extreme violence as a way of exerting sexual dominance and control over their victims. Sexual sadists often harbor deviant sexual fantasies in which they fantasize about dominating and controlling others through violence. In the case of Jack the Ripper, his crimes suggest that he may have used violence and mutilation as a way to assert his dominance over women, particularly prostitutes, whom he may have viewed as subservient or degraded in the social hierarchy. By killing and mutilating these women, the Ripper may have been acting out deep-seated fantasies of control and submission, deriving psychological and possibly sexual gratification from the act of subjugating his victims.

While Jack the Ripper's behavior is largely consistent with psychopathy and sexual sadism, some psychologists and criminologists have speculated that he may have also suffered from **paranoid delusions** or **psychotic episodes**. This would suggest a more severe form of mental illness, possibly involving schizophrenia or another psychotic disorder. The sheer brutality of the Ripper's crimes, combined with the fact that he carried out such grotesque acts in public spaces, raises questions about his level of rationality. While the mutilations were often precise, they were also reckless and overt, suggesting a level of disorganized thinking that is characteristic of individuals experiencing psychosis. For example, some of the victims were left in highly visible locations, and the mutilations were carried out with such ferocity that they suggest a loss of control or a break with reality. These behaviors could indicate that Jack the Ripper was experiencing a psychotic break, where his actions were driven by irrational impulses rather than calculated logic. It is possible that Jack the Ripper harbored paranoid delusions, believing that he was being persecuted by society or that he was on a divine or grandiose mission. Serial killers with paranoid delusions often justify their actions through warped beliefs, viewing their victims as representatives of a persecutory force or as symbolic targets in a larger mission. For example, the Ripper may have believed that prostitutes represented a societal ill that needed to be eradicated, justifying his violence as a form of purification or punishment. Alternatively, he may have seen himself as a grand figure acting on divine or supernatural orders, thus removing any sense of guilt or accountability.

Understanding Jack the Ripper's psychological profile requires a consideration of the social and environmental context in which he operated. Whitechapel in the late 19th century was a densely populated, poverty-stricken area plagued by crime, disease, and overcrowding. The social conditions of the time likely contributed to the Ripper's ability to blend into the background and exploit vulnerable women who had little protection or social support. It is possible that Jack the Ripper's motivations were influenced by a sense of frustration and alienation stemming from his social standing. Many serial killers have been found to harbor deep resentments toward society, particularly when they perceive themselves as marginalized or powerless. In the context of late 19th-century London, the Ripper may have been a working-class man who felt overlooked or powerless in the rigid social hierarchy of the time. His choice of victims—prostitutes—may have been a reflection of his disdain for women whom he viewed as morally corrupt or representative of the social decay around him. The extreme violence exhibited in the Ripper's crimes may have been a way for him to express his feelings of powerlessness and assert control in a society where he felt marginalized. By targeting vulnerable women, he may have been acting out his frustrations and using violence as a means of compensating for feelings of inadequacy or lack of control in other areas of his life.

Jack the Ripper's desire for recognition and his taunting of the police through letters suggest traits of **Narcissistic Personality Disorder (NPD)**. Narcissistic individuals often have an inflated sense of self-importance and crave admiration, sometimes even seeking notoriety through criminal acts. The letters sent to the police, including the infamous "From Hell" letter, suggest that the Ripper derived a sense of satisfaction from outsmarting the authorities and basking in the public fear he created.

The public nature of the Ripper's crimes, combined with the letters he allegedly sent to the police, suggests a desire for recognition. Narcissistic individuals often crave attention and admiration, and the Ripper's actions can be viewed as an attempt to create a public persona that would instill fear and awe. His taunts to the police indicate that he enjoyed the notoriety and believed himself to be superior to the law enforcement officials tasked with capturing him.

This sense of grandiosity is a hallmark of NPD, where individuals often overestimate their own abilities and seek to be the center of attention, even through criminal means. Narcissistic individuals often lack empathy and view others as tools to be exploited for their own gain. In the case of Jack the Ripper, his victims were likely seen as nothing more than means to an end—objects to be used in his quest for dominance and recognition. His lack of empathy for the suffering he caused is consistent with the emotional detachment seen in individuals with NPD, who are often unable or unwilling to consider the impact of their actions on others.

Possible Treatment

In the context of the late 19th century, effective treatment for an individual like Jack the Ripper would have been virtually nonexistent. Today, a person displaying similar behavior might be diagnosed with severe antisocial personality disorder, possibly combined with a paraphilic disorder involving sexual sadism (Hickey, 2016).

Modern therapeutic approaches could include cognitive-behavioral therapy (CBT) to address maladaptive thought patterns and behaviors, though the effectiveness of such treatments on individuals with profound antisocial tendencies is limited. Medications might be used to manage comorbid conditions such as psychosis or severe mood disorders, but there is no pharmacological solution for the underlying personality pathology (Hare, 1999).

Captivation and Trial

Numerous suspects have been proposed over the years, ranging from local butchers and doctors to members of the British royal family. However, the lack of concrete evidence and the limitations of forensic science at the time prevented the conclusive identification and capture of the Ripper (Evans & Rumbelow, 2006).

Conclusion

Jack the Ripper's case remains one of the most enduring mysteries in criminal history. His ability to evade capture and the enduring fascination with his crimes highlight the complexities of criminal behavior and the challenges faced by early law enforcement agencies. Studying the Ripper's psychological profile offers valuable insights into the mind of a serial killer and underscores the importance of advancements in forensic science and criminal psychology.

References

Begg, P. (2013). *Jack the Ripper: The definitive history*. Routledge.
Cook, A. (2009). *Jack the Ripper: Case closed*. Amberley Publishing.
Douglas, J., & Olshaker, M. (1997). *Mindhunter: Inside the FBI's elite serial crime unit*. Scribner.
Evans, S., & Rumbelow, D. (2006). *Jack the Ripper: Scotland Yard investigates*. Sutton Publishing.
Hare, R. D. (1999). *Without conscience: The disturbing world of the psychopaths among us*. Guilford Press.
Hickey, E. W. (2016). *Serial murderers and their victims* (7th ed.). Cengage Learning.
Keppel, R. D., Weis, J. G., Brown, K. M., & Welch, K. (2005). The Jack the Ripper murders: A modus operandi and signature analysis of the 1888–1891 Whitechapel murders. *Journal of Investigative Psychology and Offender Profiling*, 2(1), 1–21. https://doi.org/10.1002/jip.22
Rumbelow, D. (2004). *The complete Jack the Ripper*. Penguin Books.

5

THE MARC DUTROUX CASE

Introduction

Marc Dutroux, a Belgian serial killer, rapist, and child molester, became infamous for his heinous crimes against young girls in the mid-1990s. His case revealed shocking failures in the Belgian legal and law enforcement systems, leading to widespread public outrage and significant reforms (Cohen, 1997). This case study explores Dutroux's background, criminal behavior, psychological profile, possible treatment, captivation, trial, and the aftermath of his crimes.

Marc Dutroux's case is one of the most disturbing and significant in the annals of criminal psychology. His gruesome actions not only shed light on the mind of a deeply disturbed individual but also exposed systemic flaws in the institutions meant to protect society's most vulnerable members. This study examines the multifaceted aspects of Dutroux's crimes and their broader implications.

Background

Dutroux was born on November 6, 1956, in Ixelles, Brussels. He was the eldest of five children in a family where his parents were both educators. Reports indicate that he experienced physical abuse during childhood, which may have influenced his later violent tendencies. The role of genetics in criminal behavior is an area of ongoing research; however, some studies suggest that certain genetic predispositions may increase the likelihood of antisocial behavior (Donahue, 2023).

DOI: 10.4324/9781003602927-7

As an adult Dutroux moved from place to place, working as an electrician and, allegedly, a sex worker. Gradually, he turned to a life of crime—dealing drugs, stealing and trading stolen cars, and mugging. Allegedly, he amassed enough money doing this that he eventually owned seven houses (Donahue, 2023).

Dutroux was married by the time he was 20 and had two sons. His first wife would later claim that Dutroux had beaten her and had multiple extramarital affairs. The two separated in the early 1980s, leaving Dutroux free to pursue one of the women with whom he had had an affair: Michelle Martin. Martin was his second wife and also an accomplice in his crimes (Cohen, 1997).

In the summer of 1985, Marc Dutroux reportedly grew increasingly frustrated with the perceived difficulty of engaging with women and subsequently resorted to abducting and sexually assaulting them, enlisting the assistance of his second wife in these criminal actions. Later, his family friend Jean Van Peteghem also joined the couple. The pattern of crime remained the same in all the kidnappings and rapes. They targeted a lone girl walking all by herself, grabbed her or treated her and then pulled her into a van. They took the victim to his house and raped her. Dutroux even filmed them and then once done they would release them in their neighborhood.

Neurobiological factors also warrant consideration. Research has indicated that brain abnormalities can be linked to violent behavior. While specific studies on Dutroux's neurobiology are lacking, it is plausible that he may have exhibited traits associated with psychopathy—characterized by a lack of empathy, impulsivity, and manipulative behaviors. These traits are often observed in serial offenders and could explain their capacity for extreme violence without remorse (Bannon, Salis, & O'Leary, 2015).

Dutroux operated within a socio-economic context characterized by significant social stratification and urban decay. Born in Ixelles, Brussels, he grew up in a family where educational values were emphasized; however, his experiences of familial abuse and neglect likely contributed to his eventual deviance (Cohen, 1997). The breakdown of family structures often correlates with increased rates of delinquency and criminal behavior. Research indicates that children from unstable family environments are at higher risk for future criminal involvement due to a lack of social support and guidance.

In the late 20th century, Belgium was experiencing economic challenges, including unemployment and social unrest. These factors can create an environment where crime flourishes, particularly in marginalized communities. Dutroux's criminal enterprises—ranging from auto theft to child abduction—thrived in this context of economic desperation and social disillusionment. His ability to manipulate the system and exploit vulnerable individuals reflects a broader societal failure to protect at-risk populations.

Criminal Behavior

Dutroux's criminal activities began in the 1980s with a series of thefts, burglaries, and carjackings. He was first convicted of kidnapping and raping young girls in 1989 but was released on parole after serving just 3 years of his 13-year sentence. This early release set the stage for his later, more horrific crimes (Lalieu, 2004).

Between 1995 and 1996, Dutroux kidnapped, raped, and murdered several young girls. His modus operandi involved abducting girls, often with the help of his wife, Michelle Martin, and accomplice Michel Lelièvre. Dutroux would imprison his victims in a specially constructed dungeon in his basement, where they were subjected to prolonged abuse (Bourlet, 2004).

Dutroux's crimes were marked by extreme brutality and meticulous planning. He used drugs to subdue his victims and constructed soundproof cells to prevent their cries for help from being heard. The discovery of the bodies of two girls, Julie Lejeune and Melissa Russo, in his dungeon highlighted the sheer horror of his actions and the tragic fate of his victims (Frey, 2006).

> Dutroux's wife, Michele Martin, a former primary school teacher and the mother of his three children, has admitted that, in 1995, she knew two small girls were incarcerated without food or water in a secret dungeon in the cellar of a house they owned in Charleroi. She told police she visited the house to feed their dogs while her husband was in jail on car-theft charges, but she was "too frightened" to feed the girls.
>
> *(Reporter, 2020)*

Psychological Profile

A combination of severe personality disorders and psychopathic traits characterizes Marc Dutroux's psychological profile. He exhibited signs of antisocial personality disorder, including a lack of empathy, manipulativeness, and a propensity for violent behavior. His actions also suggest elements of narcissistic personality disorder, with a grandiose sense of self-importance and a need for admiration (Gordon, 2001).

Dutroux's paraphilic interests, particularly pedophilia, were central to his criminal behavior. His meticulous planning and the construction of a hidden dungeon indicate a high level of premeditation and a disturbing level of commitment to his deviant desires. Dutroux's ability to maintain a facade of normalcy while committing such heinous acts underscores the complexity of his psychological makeup (Frey, 2006).

The Marc Dutroux case remains one of the most disturbing examples of violent criminal behavior, encompassing kidnapping, sexual assault, torture, and murder. Dutroux, a Belgian serial killer active in the 1980s and 1990s, is responsible for the abduction and abuse of multiple young girls, several of whom were ultimately killed (Cohen, 1997). His psychological profile provides insight into a deeply disturbed mind characterized by psychopathy, sadistic tendencies, and sexual deviance, coupled with a highly manipulative and exploitative nature. This profile aims to unpack the key aspects of Dutroux's personality and motivations, providing an analysis rooted in forensic psychology.

Psychopathy is a personality disorder marked by a lack of empathy, remorse, and conscience, accompanied by manipulative and often violent behavior. Individuals with antisocial personality disorder (ASPD) are known for their disregard for social norms and the rights of others, and Dutroux's behavior exemplifies these traits (Hare, 1999). Throughout his criminal career, Dutroux displayed a complete lack of empathy for his victims, treating them as objects rather than human beings. His calm demeanor in court and lack of remorse reflect the emotional detachment typical of psychopathy.

Dutroux showed signs of grandiosity, another hallmark of psychopathy, by believing himself to be immune to consequences. He was manipulative, coercing others to assist him, including his wife and accomplice, Michelle Martin. This manipulative behavior allowed him to deceive those around him and evade capture despite prior arrests for similar offenses. He convinced his accomplices to engage in horrific crimes, including the abduction and imprisonment of young girls. His ability to control others and instill fear in his victims illustrates the typical psychopathic drive for power and dominance. Despite multiple arrests and convictions, Dutroux's crimes continued, highlighting his disregard for legal authority. His behavior demonstrates a fundamental lack of conscience and respect for social rules, consistent with ASPD. Even after serving time in prison, Dutroux continued his crimes upon release, undeterred by any potential consequences. He engaged in kidnapping and sexual exploitation with apparent indifference to societal norms and laws, reflecting a deeply ingrained antisocial personality.

A key component of Dutroux's psychological profile is his sadistic personality. Sadism is marked by deriving pleasure from the pain and suffering of others, and Dutroux's behavior shows clear sadistic tendencies. His crimes involved not only kidnapping and sexual assault but also prolonged psychological and physical torture of his victims. Dutroux's willingness to imprison and starve his victims, even leading to their deaths, suggests a drive to assert total control over others' lives, relishing in the power he held over his victims' survival. Dutroux's crimes indicate the presence of paraphilic disorders, specifically pedophilia and sexual sadism. Pedophilia, or the sexual attraction to prepubescent children, appears to have been a driving force in his selection of young female victims. His sadistic tendencies compounded this deviance, as he sought to derive pleasure from the domination and suffering of vulnerable children. His behavior aligns with sexually sadistic offenders who derive pleasure from both sexual gratification and the psychological impact of instilling fear and pain.

Paraphilic disorders like pedophilia are challenging to treat and often lead to escalating behaviors, as seen in Dutroux's progression from sexual assault to murder. The combination of these disorders created a pattern in which Dutroux's deviant desires led to repeated, increasingly brutal offenses, each escalating in terms of violence and psychological torment inflicted on his victims.

Dutroux exhibited strong narcissistic traits, manifesting as a need for admiration, sense of entitlement, and obsession with control. Narcissistic individuals often have an inflated sense of self-importance and believe they are entitled to exploit others. Dutroux displayed these traits by viewing his victims as his property, objects to be controlled and disposed of at his will. His elaborate plans for abduction, construction of underground prison cells, and calculated steps to evade detection show a meticulous need for control, which is typical in narcissistic offenders who view others as mere tools for their own satisfaction. Dutroux's narcissism also fueled his need for recognition. His belief in his own superiority led him to manipulate those around him, assuming that he was beyond reproach and untouchable. This entitlement made him take risks and continue his criminal behavior despite being under police scrutiny, further underscoring the grandiosity associated with narcissistic personality traits.

Despite his various relationships and accomplices, Dutroux's connections with others were transactional and devoid of true emotional bonds. Psychopathic individuals are often incapable of forming authentic attachments, and Dutroux's relationships were marked by manipulation and exploitation. His accomplice and wife, Michelle Martin, was coerced into assisting him, yet he treated her merely as a tool for achieving his own ends. His interactions with his victims, devoid of empathy or compassion, further highlight his inability to connect with others on a human level.

Some theorists argue that Dutroux may have harbored feelings of inadequacy or alienation, which contributed to his violent behavior. Criminals with psychopathic tendencies often have backgrounds marked by neglect or abuse, though it is not confirmed if Dutroux experienced this. Regardless, Dutroux's actions suggest a deep-seated resentment toward society and an urge to assert his power, potentially compensating for underlying feelings of alienation or inferiority. His choice of young, vulnerable victims who could not resist or fight back allowed Dutroux to feel dominant and in control, offering him a twisted sense of validation and power. This behavior aligns with criminal profiling insights, suggesting that offenders often choose victims who represent societal vulnerabilities, thereby allowing them to project their own resentments.

Marc Dutroux's psychological profile is a chilling blend of psychopathy, sexual sadism, narcissism, and severe paraphilic disorders. His lack of empathy, manipulation of others, and desire for power reveal a deeply disturbed individual who found satisfaction in the suffering and subjugation of others. His crimes were not only acts of violence but carefully orchestrated expressions of control, driven by a profound need to dominate and degrade. Dutroux's case highlights the dangers of unchecked psychopathy and underscores the need for vigilance in managing individuals with such severe psychological disorders. His behavior exemplifies the tragic intersection of mental illness and criminality, revealing a mind consumed by deviant desires and a complete disregard for human life. Understanding Dutroux's psychological profile offers a cautionary perspective on the complexities of violent offenders and the importance of comprehensive psychological evaluation and intervention in preventing similar tragedies.

Possible Treatment

Treating an individual with Marc Dutroux's psychological profile would be an extraordinarily complex and challenging task. His combination of antisocial and narcissistic personality disorders, coupled with paraphilic interests, would likely resist conventional therapeutic interventions.

Cognitive-behavioral therapy (CBT) might address some of his cognitive distortions and maladaptive thought patterns, but its effectiveness would be limited due to the depth and severity of his disorders. Additionally, his lack of empathy and remorse, characteristic of psychopathy, would pose significant barriers to successful treatment (Hare, 1999).

Medications might be used to manage comorbid conditions such as depression or anxiety, but there is no pharmacological treatment for the underlying personality pathology. Long-term incarceration and isolation would likely remain the most effective way to manage the risk he poses to society (Stone, 2001).

Captivation and Trial

Marc Dutroux was apprehended in August 1996 after one of his accomplices, Michel Lelièvre, was arrested and led the police to Dutroux's residence. The discovery of the imprisoned girls and the bodies of his victims in Dutroux's properties shocked the nation and led to a massive investigation (Bourlet, 2004).

Dutroux's trial began in 2004, 8 years after his arrest, due to extensive delays and procedural issues. During the trial, Dutroux displayed no remorse and attempted to shift blame onto his accomplices and the authorities. He was ultimately convicted of multiple charges, including murder, kidnapping, and rape, and was sentenced to life imprisonment (Lalieu, 2004).

Conclusion

The case of Marc Dutroux remains one of the most harrowing examples of serial crime in modern history. His actions not only devastated the lives of his victims and their families but also exposed deep flaws in the Belgian criminal justice system. Studying Dutroux's psychological profile and criminal behavior provides valuable insights into the mind of a serial predator and underscores the importance of robust legal and protective measures to prevent such tragedies in the future.

References

Bannon, S. M., Salis, K. L., & O'Leary, K. D. (2015). Structural brain abnormalities in aggression and violent behavior. *Aggression and Violent Behavior*, *25*, 323–331. https://doi.org/10.1016/j.avb.2015.09.016

Bourlet, J. (2004). *Marc Dutroux: The hidden horror*. Presses Universitaires de France.

Cohen, R. (1997, November 3). A new set of killings deepens Belgium's darkness. *The New York Times*. https://www.nytimes.com/1997/11/03/world/a-new-set-of-killings-deepens-belgium-s-darkness.html

Donahue, M. (2023, October 13). Marc Dutroux, the killer who built a "House of horror" in Belgium. *All That's Interesting*. https://allthatsinteresting.com/marc-dutroux

Frey, H. (2006). *The Dutroux affair: Belgium's modern tragedy*. Leuven University Press.

Gordon, J. (2001). *Personality disorders in modern criminal psychology*. Routledge.

Hare, R. D. (1999). *Without conscience: The disturbing world of the psychopaths among us*. Guilford Press.

Lalieu, M. (2004). *The Dutroux case: A legal and psychological examination*. Wolters Kluwer.

Reporter, G. S. (2020, July 16). Belgium's silent heart of darkness. *The Guardian*. https://www.theguardian.com/world/2002/may/05/dutroux.featuresreview

Stone, M. H. (2001). Serial killers: An epidemiological study of their mental disorders. *American Journal of Psychiatry*, *158*(6), 903–908.

6

CASE STUDY ON ORENTHAL JAMES SIMPSON

Introduction

The Orenthal James Simpson (O. J. Simpson) trial, often dubbed the "Trial of the Century," captivated public attention and legal experts worldwide. This case was one of the most tumultuous as Simpson went from football Hall of Famer to movie star to double murder suspect. O. J. Simpson was charged with the brutal murder of his ex-wife, her friend, and a waiter. Three decades later, the infamous crime remains unsolved (Marcia, 1996). This case study delves into the trial's significance, exploring the psychological and forensic dimensions, as well as its broader implications for the legal system.

Background

Athlete and actor O. J. Simpson was born on July 9, 1947, in San Francisco, California. He was the youngest of his four siblings. He grew up in a single-parent household, with his mother being the sole breadwinner of the family. Simpson was diagnosed with rickets when he was 2 years old and had to wear leg braces till he was 13, which led to him being teased around during his childhood. Around his teenage years, he had a fair share of run-ins with the law (Warren, 2019).

His early life was marked by various challenges, including academic difficulties and behavioral issues, which prevented him from securing college scholarship offers while in high school. Despite these setbacks, Simpson demonstrated exceptional athletic prowess, especially after setting multiple junior college records. His performance ultimately attracted the attention of

DOI: 10.4324/9781003602927-8

university recruiters, earning him a scholarship to the University of Southern California (USC), where he joined the football team (Cahill, 2024).

During his second season at USC, Simpson achieved significant success, setting NCAA records for rushing yards in a season (1,709) and total carries (355), contributing to the team's national championship victory. His remarkable achievements culminated in him winning the prestigious 1968 Heisman Trophy by a record margin (Reyes, 2024).

Simpson's professional football career began when he was selected as the first overall pick by the Buffalo Bills in the 1969 NFL Draft. Although his first three seasons in the NFL were relatively uneventful, his talent eventually became undeniable. In 1972, Simpson led the NFL in rushing for four out of five seasons until 1976. In 1973, he made history by becoming the first NFL player to rush over 2,000 yards in a 14-game season, earning him the NFL Most Valuable Player (MVP) award (Reyes, 2024).

Parallel to his sports career, Simpson pursued acting, debuting in the television series Medical Center while negotiating his contract with the Buffalo Bills. He later appeared in the celebrated miniseries *Roots* (1977) and in films such as *The Towering Inferno* (1974), *The Cassandra Crossing* (1976), *Capricorn One* (1977), and the *Naked Gun* film series (1988, 1991, 1994) (Cahill, 2024).

During the trail sessions, A judge Jackie Glass said

> Earlier in this case, at a bail hearing, I asked, I said, to Mr. Simpson, I didn't know if he was arrogant or ignorant or both. And during the trial and through this proceeding, I got this answer, and it was both.

Later his arrogance and ignorance could also be understood by the way he wrote a detailed description on how he would kill his wife and a few others if given a change in his book titled "If I Did It," which was to be published by FOX publication. However, the scheduled publisher terminated the controversial project following widespread public outrage over the book deal (Marcia, 1996).

O. J. Simpson was charged with the brutal murders of his ex-wife, Nicole Brown Simpson, and her friend, Ronald Goldman, in June 1994. The subsequent trial, which commenced in January 1995, became a media sensation, reflecting deep-seated public interest and controversy. The case was marked by its unprecedented media coverage and sensationalism, reflecting broader societal issues, including race and celebrity culture (Dershowitz, 1996; Marcia, 1996).

The prosecution's case was built around compelling DNA evidence, witness testimonies, and Simpson's documented history of domestic violence. In contrast, Simpson's defense team, led by the renowned attorney Johnnie

Cochran, mounted a vigorous challenge against the prosecution's evidence, arguing that it had been mishandled and suggesting that Simpson was a victim of racial bias and police misconduct (Kunstler, 1997; Murphy, 1995).

The trial's media frenzy contributed to its status as a defining moment in American legal history, highlighting the profound effects of media on public perception and the justice system (Tushnet, 1998). The trial's backdrop was also marked by racial tensions and high-profile personalities, which further amplified its dramatic impact on the national consciousness.

Criminal Behavior

The prosecution contended that Simpson acted out of jealousy and rage, presenting a combination of DNA evidence, witness accounts, and Simpson's history of abusive behavior toward Nicole Brown Simpson. However, Simpson's defense team argued that the evidence was not only mishandled but also tainted by racial prejudice. High-profile lawyer Johnnie Cochran famously argued that Simpson was being framed by the Los Angeles Police Department (LAPD), a strategy that resonated with many observers and contributed to the trial's dramatic nature (Kunstler, 1997).

The Simpson case can be considered as a classic example of the tragic end of a tumultuous relationship riddled with intimate partner violence. There were many reports of Simpson's violence toward Brown throughout the course of their marriage. Spousal battery charges were finally filed in 1989, and it was not till 1992 that they formally divorced. In 1993, they got back together for a brief period of time; however, Simpson reverted to his old ways after getting to know about the relationship Brown had during the time they had separated. Brown ended their relationship for good post this incident.

Nicole Brown and her friend Ron Goldman were found stabbed to death outside Brown's apartment complex. She was found lying in a fetal position with seven stab wounds on her neck and scalp. The wounds were so deep that she was almost decapitated (Guerrasio, 2016). Goldman had multiple stab wounds to his torso and a fatal wound to his neck. He also had aberrations on his knuckles, indicating defensive wounds (Jack Walraven's Simpson Trial Transcripts, n.d.). Though Simpson have been acquitted of the criminal charges, he was held liable for the civil charges on the wrongful deaths of Brown and Goldman (Simon, 1997).

Following his acquittal, Simpson was involved in multiple criminal charges on multiple occasions, including battery, drug possession, tax evasion, money laundering, etc. He has neither been charged nor been acquitted in all the above cases. Simpson was also a part of an equally infamous armed robbery, for which he served 9 years in prison. He had broken and entered a casino in 2007 and stolen sports memorabilia with three other men (Burke, 2024).

Psychological Profile

In examining Simpson's psychological profile, evaluations revealed traits consistent with narcissistic personality disorder (NPD), such as a grandiose sense of self-importance and difficulties in managing interpersonal relationships and emotions. The prosecution highlighted the influence of jealousy and a history of domestic violence as contributing factors to the alleged crimes. Psychological analyses provided insights into Simpson's motivations, including the potential role of narcissistic tendencies in his actions (Millon, Simonsen, Birket-Smith, & Davis, 2010; Smith & Johnson, 2005).

O. J. Simpson, a former football star and actor, was famously tried for the murder of his ex-wife Nicole Brown Simpson and her friend Ron Goldman in 1994 (Burke, 2024). Although he was acquitted in the criminal trial, a civil court later found him liable for their wrongful deaths. Analyzing his psychological profile requires a careful examination of his personality traits, relationship dynamics, and potential psychological factors that may have contributed to the alleged crime. This psychological profile is drawn from public records, trial evidence, interviews, and analyses by mental health professionals who have speculated on his psychological state based on available information.

O. J. Simpson's early life and rise to fame play a key role in understanding his psychological makeup. Growing up in a challenging environment, Simpson experienced poverty and family struggles, which arguably fostered a strong drive for success and social status. He compensated for these early hardships with outstanding athletic achievements, eventually reaching fame as an NFL player. His successful career afforded him not only wealth and public adoration but also a sense of invincibility and entitlement. This entitlement may have shaped his perception of relationships and behavior, reinforcing his belief that he was above reproach.

Simpson's personality traits also seem to reflect characteristics consistent with NPD. NPD is often characterized by an exaggerated sense of self-importance, a need for excessive admiration, a lack of empathy, and difficulties in handling criticism. Simpson exhibited many behaviors suggestive of these traits, such as grandiosity, an expectation of preferential treatment, and extreme reactions to perceived slights. His image in the public eye, coupled with his athletic and celebrity status, could have fueled his narcissistic tendencies, reinforcing a self-image where he was in control and admired. Additionally, his interactions with Nicole Brown suggested a possessive and controlling attitude, which may have stemmed from his need to maintain dominance in personal relationships.

O. J. Simpson's relationship with Nicole Brown was tumultuous and marked by instances of violence, jealousy, and control. Their marriage was marred by numerous reports of domestic abuse, with police records showing multiple incidents where Brown reported being physically assaulted by

Simpson. This pattern of violence suggests a combination of power and possessiveness, qualities often seen in individuals who view relationships as extensions of their self-image. Simpson's aggression toward Brown likely stemmed from feelings of ownership and a deep-seated need to control her actions and choices, which he may have seen as reflections of his own self-worth and authority.

Jealousy and possessiveness are common in relationships where one partner feels entitled to dominate the other. Simpson's behavior toward Brown indicates that he struggled with feelings of jealousy and suspicion, especially after their divorce. His inability to let go of control may have been compounded by a belief that Brown's choices reflected on him personally, which might have fueled his anger and resentment toward her. Reports suggest that Simpson continued to monitor and interact with Brown in controlling ways even after their divorce, perhaps feeling that she had violated his sense of ownership by seeking independence.

Several psychological factors might have contributed to Simpson's alleged actions against Nicole Brown. First, his behavior aligns with characteristics seen in narcissistic rage—a term used to describe intense outbursts or violent reactions from individuals with narcissistic traits when they perceive a threat to their self-image or control. Brown's attempts to distance herself from Simpson may have triggered such rage, with Simpson feeling that her actions represented a personal betrayal or rejection. This perception could have escalated into violence, particularly if Simpson felt that his public persona or self-worth was threatened by the end of their relationship.

Additionally, Simpson may have experienced borderline personality features, particularly in his relationships and emotional responses. Borderline personality disorder (BPD) is marked by intense, unstable relationships and emotional dysregulation, often resulting in impulsive and extreme reactions. Although not formally diagnosed, individuals exhibiting borderline characteristics can experience intense abandonment fears and difficulty coping with relationship losses, sometimes reacting with extreme anger or aggression. Simpson's inability to move on from Brown, combined with his history of emotional volatility, suggests that he might have struggled with an unstable self-image tied to his relationships, leading to potential impulsivity and aggression.

The stress of public scrutiny, combined with his struggle to maintain control over his image, could have also contributed to Simpson's mental state. Public figures often experience immense pressure to uphold their reputations, and Simpson was particularly attuned to his public image. For individuals with narcissistic or controlling tendencies, perceived public humiliation can be profoundly threatening. The end of his marriage to Brown and her independence may have represented not only personal loss but also public rejection, a situation he may have found intolerable given his established image.

O. J. Simpson's environment likely played a role in shaping his behavior and attitudes. As a celebrated athlete and public figure, Simpson was accustomed to preferential treatment and a level of respect and authority rarely questioned. This environment may have reinforced his sense of entitlement and reduced his capacity to cope with frustration or rejection. Simpson's status as a celebrity meant that he was frequently insulated from the consequences of his actions, including his alleged abuse of Brown. This insulation may have contributed to his belief that he was exempt from accountability, reinforcing a pattern of dominating and controlling behavior that ultimately culminated in the tragic events of 1994.

Furthermore, societal expectations and cultural attitudes toward male dominance in relationships may have influenced Simpson's perceptions of power and control. Simpson emerged from a generation where masculinity was often associated with dominance, aggression, and control over family matters, attitudes that could have shaped his view of his relationship with Brown. As Brown attempted to assert her independence, Simpson may have perceived this as a challenge to his traditional role and authority, further fueling his possessiveness and aggression.

O. J. Simpson's alleged actions toward Nicole Brown were likely the result of a complex interplay between his narcissistic personality traits, emotional instability, and inability to cope with perceived threats to his self-image and control. His background, personality characteristics, and history of violence indicate a pattern of behavior consistent with controlling and potentially violent individuals. Simpson's need to assert dominance and maintain his self-image likely fueled his inability to let go of Brown and contributed to a psychological environment in which he saw violence as a means to regain control. The tragedy surrounding this case underscores how deeply entrenched personality traits, coupled with societal influences and personal insecurities, can culminate in actions that harm others in profoundly irreversible ways.

Ultimately, understanding O. J. Simpson's psychological profile may provide insight into how personality traits, environmental influences, and emotional triggers can interact, sometimes leading to tragic outcomes. Although many factors remain speculative, this analysis underscores the importance of addressing personality disorders, emotional dysregulation, and societal reinforcement of harmful behaviors in preventing future tragedies of similar nature.

Forensic Aspects

The forensic evidence presented in the case included advanced DNA analysis, crime scene reconstructions, and expert testimonies. The trial underscored the challenges of conveying complex forensic evidence to a jury, as well as the substantial impact of media coverage on public opinion and the judicial process. The defense's strategy to undermine forensic credibility and accuse the police of racial bias played a crucial role in shaping the trial's outcome and public discourse (Kunstler, 1997; Turner, 2001).

Captivation and Trial

The trials of the O. J. Simpson case were marred by media sensationalism and legal irregularities. Simpson's acquittal in October 1995 was a landmark verdict that sparked intense debates about race, justice, and the role of media in legal proceedings. The trial exposed the profound influence of the media on legal outcomes and the challenges of ensuring an impartial jury in high-profile cases. The case remains a focal point for discussions on the effectiveness of forensic evidence and the impact of public opinion on legal decisions (Dershowitz, 1996; Tushnet, 1998).

The prosecution had a large proportion of physical evidence including bloody footprints in the crime scene that matched Simpson, hair samples at the scene of crime, Simpson's blood sample from the crime scene. However, the improper management of the evidence by the LAPD gave the defense team enough leverage. They argued that the officers who handled the case were racist and had framed Simpson. The jury acquitted Simpson of all his charges after a months-long trial. He was, however, held liable in a civil case about the wrongful deaths of Brown and Goldman (Kunstler, 1997).

Conclusion

The O. J. Simpson trial remains a landmark case in legal history, offering critical insights into the interplay of psychology, forensic evidence, and media influence. Its enduring impact on public perceptions of justice and race continues to shape discussions about the legal system.

References

Burke, L. V. (2024, April 18). *Football legend O.J. Simpson dies, but the obsession remains alive*. The Seattle Medium. https://seattlemedium.com/football-legend-o-j-simpson-dies-but-the-obsession-remains-alive/

Cahill, T. (2024, April 11). O.J. Simpson: A man for offseason. *Rolling Stone*. https://www.rollingstone.com/culture/culture-sports/o-j-simpson-a-man-for-offseason-186994/

Dershowitz, A. (1996). *The best defense*. Random House.

Guerrasio, J. (2016, June 16). ESPN is showing horrific never-before-seen murder photos in its new O.J. Simpson documentary. *Business Insider India*. https://www.businessinsider.in/espn-is-showing-horrific-never-before-seen-murder-photos-in-its-new-o-j-simpson-documentary/articleshow/52782897.cms

Jack Walraven's Simpson Trial Transcripts. (n.d.). https://simpson.walraven.org/autop-rg.html

Kunstler, W. M. (1997). *The defense never rests*. HarperCollins.
Marcia, S. (1996). *The O.J. Simpson case: The people versus O.J.* Simpson. New York Review of Books.
Millon, T., Simonsen, E., Birket-Smith, M., & Davis, R. D. (2010). *Psychopathy: Antisocial, criminal, and violent behavior* (2nd ed.). Guilford Press.
Murphy, K. (1995). *The trial of O.J. Simpson: A social and legal history*. Routledge.
Reyes, L. (2024, April 11). Here's a look at O.J. Simpson's career highlights in football and athletics. *USA Today*. https://www.usatoday.com/story/sports/nfl/2024/04/11/oj-simpson-football-career-highlights/73290477007/
Simon, S. (1997, February 11). Simpson verdict: $25 million: Punitive damages bring total to $33.5 million. *Los Angeles Times*. https://www.latimes.com/archives/la-xpm-1997-02-11-mn-27600-story.html.
Smith, J., & Johnson, L. (2005). Narcissistic personality disorder in criminal behavior. *Psychological Bulletin*, *131*(6), 901–914.
Turner, C. (2001). Forensic science in the O.J. Simpson case: Analyzing the evidence. *Journal of Forensic Sciences*, *46*(4), 845–852.
Tushnet, M. (1998). The O.J. Simpson case and the impact of media. *Yale Law Journal*, *107*(7), 1741–1765.
Warren, J. (2019, March 14). THE SIMPSON MURDER CASE: 'I Was Somebody Who Didn't Care about Anything': Childhood: The football hero grew up in a bleak housing project in San Francisco and was often in trouble. But a jailhouse visit by baseball star Willie Mays helped the youth turn his life around. *Los Angeles Times*. https://www.latimes.com/archives/la-xpm-1994-06-18-mn-5414-story.html

7

CASE STUDY ON ANDREI CHIKATILO

Introduction

Andrei Chikatilo, one of Russia's most infamous serial killers, terrorized the Soviet Union with a series of brutal murders from 1978 to 1990. Dubbed the "Butcher of Rostov," "The Rostov Ripper," and the "The Red Ripper," Chikatilo's case exemplifies extreme psychopathy and its profound impact on criminal behavior (Cullen, 1993).

Background

Andrei Romanovich Chikatilo was born on October 16, 1936, in Yabluchne, Ukraine. His early life was marred by severe poverty, trauma from the Soviet famine of the 1930s, and the harsh realities of World War II. These formative experiences had a profound effect on his psychological development, contributing to his later criminal behavior (Kozlov, 2000; Haines, 2001). Both of Chikatilo's parents were farmers in the collective farm under Stalin's regime. His family was so impoverished that Chikatilo claims he never had proper food till the age of 12. As a child he would also hear from his mother that he had an elder brother who was kidnapped and eaten by their neighbors. The psychiatrist who interviewed (Cullen, 1993) Chikatilo also noted prenatal developmental problems including hydrocephalus and brain lesions, which could lead to bedwetting. After his father was drafted to go for the war, he continued to share a bed with his mother. He was beaten up and scolded by his mother, due to his bedwetting. He also had a younger half-sister Tatyana, who was believed to be born as a result of the rape of his mother by German soldiers (allegedly witnessed by a young Chikatilo). His father was captured

DOI: 10.4324/9781003602927-9

by Germans during the war and was viewed as a traitor; hence the Chikatilo family was isolated and humiliated for being the family members of a traitor (Cullen, 1993).

Chikatilo was a bright student, praised by his teachers and bullied by his classmates. As an adolescent, Chikatilo found himself to be impotent and found dating experiences to be not fruitful. He was also myopic but kept it to himself as he was afraid of being bullied further because of wearing spectacles. He moved to Moscow to pursue his higher education at law at the age of 19; however, he was allegedly rejected due to his father being a "traitor." He later acquired a communications diploma and worked as a communication technician. In 1957, he was drafted to the army and worked as a communication technician (Cullen, 1993).

After being discharged from the army, he married and had two children. He also secured a degree from Rostov University in Russian literature. He later shifted his career to the education sector as the deputy director of a vocational school, but was unable to garner the respect of the students. During the course of his work he began to molest his students. He was asked to resign from his position and went on to secure a job as an educator at another vocational school. He managed to continue in this position without much incident till he was let go because of downsizing. He was able to secure a job as an instructor in another technical school where his wife also started to work. His killing sprees started during this period. Around 1981 he was reported by many students for sexual assaults and molestation. He later took up a job as a supply clerk for a factory that produced construction material (Cullen, 1993).

Chikatilo's upbringing in a war-torn region, combined with his impoverished background, shaped his worldview and personality. The trauma and deprivations of his early years are believed to have influenced his psychological and emotional development, contributing to his later manifestations of extreme violence and psychopathy (Haines, 2001).

Criminal Behavior

Chikatilo's reign of terror included the abduction, sexual assault, and murder of at least 52 victims, many of whom were children. His crimes were characterized by their brutality and a disturbing level of ritualistic behavior. Chikatilo exhibited a pattern of extreme violence and sadism, indicating a profound psychological disturbance and a deep-seated compulsion to inflict harm (Lev, 1998; Hickey, 2016).

Chikatilo was 16 year old, when he committed his first crime, when he tried to overpower and sexually assaulted a 10 year old girl who had come to visit his sister. It was not until 20 years later that he was reported to have committed rape on two of his students. He was also reported to have been engaged in voyeurism and touching his students inappropriately during this period (Conradi, 2016).

He started acting on his sexual fantasies after he moved to secure his latest job in 1978. He bought a house to act out his sexual fantasies, starting out with soliciting prostitutes. He killed his first victim, a 9-year-old girl named Yelena Zakotnova in 1978. He had coaxed her into his hut and tried to sexually assault her. He was not able to perform sexually, which led to him stabbing her three times in her stomach, killing her in the process. Another habitual sex offender named Aleksandr Kravchenko was convicted and executed for this crime. Chikatilo found that he was able to get sexual arousal out of the act of stabbing and murder, which led him to taking the life of 55 more people (Conradi, 2016).

His next victim was Larisa Tkachenko, a 17-year-old girl, who was strangled, beaten, and mutilated. With his next victim, 13-year-old Lyubov Biryuk, there was an escalation in the number of stabbings as Biryuk had 22 stab wounds on her body. Over time he developed a signature style of carving out the eye sockets of the victims, mutilation, and even disembowelment. In 1984, he was arrested for suspicious interaction with young women, who fitted the victim profile of the serial killer who was being searched by the police. He was let go as his blood type did not match the sample obtained from the site of the crime. He was, however, added to the list of suspects in the Rostov murder cases. He kept a low profile for a while and continued with his killings in places far from Rostov. Most of his victims were found near a railway line around Rostov Oblast. His last victim was 22-year-old Svetlana Korostik. Chikatilo, who was washing himself near a well, was spotted by an on-duty policeman who found him suspicious. This ultimately led to his capture and arrest (Conradi, 2016).

Psychological Profile

Severe psychopathic traits, including a profound lack of empathy, manipulative behavior, and a propensity for extreme violence, mark Chikatilo's psychological profile. He demonstrated characteristics of sexual sadism and antisocial personality disorder (ASPD), which fueled his violent and sadistic actions. His psychopathy was evident in his ability to evade capture for years and his calculated approach to his crimes (Hickey, 2016; Smith, 2014).

Andrei Chikatilo, known as the "Butcher of Rostov," was a Soviet serial killer who committed at least 52 murders in the 1970s and 1980s (Cullen, 1993). His brutal killings, primarily targeting women and children, left a profound psychological and cultural impact. Understanding Chikatilo's psychological profile requires an examination of his background, personality traits, interpersonal relationships, and potential psychological disorders that may have contributed to his violent behavior. His life and crimes reflect a complex interplay between environmental influences, innate personality traits, and possible neurological impairments, which together may have contributed to his extreme criminal behavior.

Born in 1936 in a small Ukrainian village during the Stalinist regime, Andrei Chikatilo's early years were marked by extreme poverty, trauma, and fear. His family faced starvation and the constant threat of violence, common experiences under the oppressive Soviet regime. Chikatilo's mother instilled in him a pervasive sense of fear, especially after his older brother was allegedly kidnapped and killed by starving villagers. This story, true or not, became a significant psychological burden for Chikatilo, shaping his worldview and self-perception (Cullen, 1993).

Chikatilo's childhood was marked by physical and emotional abuse, further compounded by a pervasive sense of inadequacy. He suffered from enuresis (bedwetting), which often led to public humiliation, and he displayed a timid and withdrawn demeanor, making him a target of ridicule and bullying by his peers. During adolescence, he discovered that he was unable to achieve an erection or sexual satisfaction through typical interactions, which contributed to feelings of shame, frustration, and powerlessness (Cullen, 1993). This inability to connect sexually or emotionally with others would later become a crucial component of his violent tendencies. Psychologically, these early experiences likely fostered an internalized rage, a need for control, and a desire to retaliate against a world he saw as harsh and rejecting.

As Chikatilo entered adulthood, his maladaptive behaviors and personality traits became more pronounced. Though he maintained a facade of a socially acceptable life by marrying and fathering two children, he struggled to establish meaningful relationships and found satisfaction only in his fantasies. Chikatilo's lack of social skills, alongside a perceived inability to live up to societal expectations, may have intensified his feelings of inadequacy and resentment.

Chikatilo's sexual deviancy became apparent when he attempted to sexually assault a girl in his twenties. Although this incident did not lead to homicide, it hinted at his latent violent tendencies and his inability to form healthy sexual attachments. Rather than fostering connection, his sexual urges were linked to aggression, frustration, and control. His first confirmed murder in 1978, that of a 9-year-old girl, was a horrifying escalation of these fantasies (Cullen, 1993). He derived sexual gratification from violence and, over time, developed a compulsion to enact similar acts repeatedly. His murders were characterized by extreme brutality, often involving stabbing, mutilation, and cannibalism, suggesting a sadistic personality with an overwhelming need for dominance and control.

Chikatilo's personality appears to align with characteristics seen in individuals with ASPD, specifically traits of sadism, lack of empathy, and a profound disregard for others. ASPD is often marked by impulsivity, superficial charm, and a persistent violation of others' rights, all traits that Chikatilo displayed in his interactions with his victims. While he was largely withdrawn in his everyday life, he meticulously selected and lured victims, displaying a calculating and premeditated approach to his crimes. This behavior reflects a level of cognitive organization that is often associated with high-functioning psychopathy, where an individual may appear ordinary on the surface but harbors violent, antisocial tendencies.

Chikatilo's psychological profile is further complicated by signs of paraphilic disorders, particularly sexual sadism and necrophilia. Sexual sadism, a condition where individuals derive pleasure from inflicting pain and suffering, likely underpinned his violent behavior. His murders involved acts of extreme physical violence, often prolonged to maximize his gratification, indicating that the pain and terror of his victims were integral to his experience. This sadistic tendency, coupled with his history of social and sexual rejection, created a perfect storm for the development of serial violence.

Neurological factors may also have contributed to Chikatilo's actions. Some mental health professionals have speculated that he may have had undiagnosed neurological impairments, such as frontal lobe dysfunction, which is sometimes linked to impulsive and violent behavior. The frontal lobe governs impulse control, decision-making, and social behavior, and dysfunction in this area has been observed in individuals with a history of violent crimes. While there is no direct evidence of brain abnormalities in Chikatilo, his impulsive, violent actions combined with his inability to empathize suggest the possibility of neurological factors contributing to his behavior. Additionally, his use of violence to compensate for his sexual impotence indicates a deeply rooted sense of inadequacy, which may have been exacerbated by neurobiological issues affecting his sense of control and self-worth.

Chikatilo's selection of vulnerable victims—primarily young women and children—reflects a pattern seen in many serial offenders. These individuals represented the innocence and defenselessness he may have simultaneously envied and resented. Through his violent acts, he exerted control over those he perceived as weaker, symbolically reversing his own history of victimization and powerlessness. His killings followed a ritualistic pattern that provided him with a sense of mastery and predictability. Each murder reaffirmed his sense of power, offering temporary relief from his underlying feelings of inadequacy and rage.

The ritualistic aspect of his killings can be further understood through the lens of obsessive-compulsive disorder (OCD) or obsessive-compulsive personality traits. Though not a formal diagnosis, Chikatilo's repetitive, ritualistic approach suggests he experienced a compulsion to reenact specific acts, deriving psychological relief from each murder. Such compulsions can create a cycle of violence, where the individual feels compelled to repeat behaviors to satisfy underlying psychological needs, escalating over time as initial acts fail to provide the same level of satisfaction.

Chikatilo's psychological profile cannot be fully understood without considering the broader sociocultural environment in which he lived. Growing up in the Soviet Union, where social constraints were rigid, and mental health resources were scarce, Chikatilo had limited access to psychological support or intervention. His outward conformity as a teacher and family man enabled him to evade suspicion and scrutiny, reflecting a society where private struggles often went unaddressed. Additionally, the Soviet regime's emphasis on secrecy and repression may have indirectly contributed to his pathology, as his deviant behaviors were largely ignored by authorities, who failed to link him to his crimes for years.

His sense of alienation, fostered by a society that emphasized collectivism over individuality, may have reinforced his violent tendencies as he struggled to reconcile his internal world with external expectations. Chikatilo's ability to blend into society, despite his brutal actions, highlights how certain cultural and systemic failures allowed him to continue his violent acts without intervention.

Andrei Chikatilo's psychological profile is a chilling example of how environmental influences, neurological factors, personality traits, and possibly mental health disorders can combine to produce violent behavior. His early trauma, sexual inadequacies, sadistic tendencies, and possible neurological impairments created a complex and dangerous psychological landscape. Lacking empathy, driven by violent compulsions, and emboldened by social alienation, Chikatilo's actions reflect a profound pathology rooted in both his life experiences and potential biological predispositions.

Understanding Chikatilo's profile offers valuable insights into the psychological mechanisms that can lead to extreme violence. His case underscores the need for comprehensive mental health interventions and social support systems to address the factors that may contribute to such destructive behaviors.

Possible Treatment

Treating Chikatilo would have been exceptionally challenging due to his severe psychopathy and sadistic tendencies. Traditional therapeutic approaches, such as cognitive-behavioral therapy (CBT), would likely have had limited success given his entrenched personality disorders and lack of remorse. Effective treatment for such severe cases often requires innovative and highly specialized approaches, which were not available during his time (Hickey, 2016; Johnson & Peters, 2013).

Captivation and Trial

Chikatilo was apprehended in 1990 after a protracted investigation fraught with numerous false leads. His trial unveiled the full extent of his horrific crimes and the complexities of his psychological profile. Convicted of 52 murders, Chikatilo was ultimately executed in 1994. The trial not only highlighted his depravity but also underscored the difficulties in investigating and prosecuting serial killers (Lev, 1998; Brown, 2000).

Chikatilo initially entered the police radar for the serial murders as early as 1984. His suspicious behavior of approaching young women, frotteurism, and his bag containing vaseline, rope, and knife led to him being planted firmly in the suspect list. Post the discovery of the remains of his last victim, the police who had seen him washing himself near the disposal site began to consider him their prime suspect. The police monitored him for six days before arresting him, and he was seen engaging in conversation with multiple young men and women. On his arrest he had wounds inflicted on his body which could be traced to being inflicted by one of his victims. His semen sample was matched to the semen sample found near many of his victims. He had confessed to 36 of the 38 murders the police had connected to him and an additional 20 that the police had no clue about. He gave gruesome details of the murders and confessed to drinking the blood and consuming the body parts of his victims (Conradi, 2016).

Chikatilo was diagnosed with borderline personality disorder. He was declared to be fit to stand the trial. He was tried for a total of 53 murders that the police could physically link him to and 5 sexual assault charges. He was placed in an iron cage throughout the trial from the angry kins of the victim. He was found guilty for 52 murders and was sentenced to death along with 86 years of imprisonment. His execution was carried out with a single gunshot wound to his head, on February 14, 1994 (Conradi, 2016).

Conclusion

The case of Andrei Chikatilo offers a chilling glimpse into the psyche of a serial killer driven by extreme psychopathy. Analyzing his psychological profile is crucial for understanding the factors that contribute to serial murder and underscores the challenges associated with treating individuals with severe personality disorders.

References

Brown, A. (2000). *The Russian serial killer: Andrei Chikatilo's reign of terror*. Palgrave Macmillan.

Conradi, P. (2016). *The Red Ripper: Inside the mind of Russia's most brutal serial killer*. Open Road Media.

Cullen, R. (1993). *The killer department: Detective Burakov's eight-year hunt for the most savage serial killer in Russian history*. Pantheon Books.
Haines, J. (2001). The impact of early trauma on criminal behavior: A case study of Andrei Chikatilo. *Journal of Forensic Sciences*, *46*(2), 456–464.
Hickey, E. W. (2016). *Serial murderers and their victims* (7th ed.). Cengage Learning.
Johnson, H., & Peters, M. (2013). Innovative approaches to treating severe psychopathy. *Behavioral Sciences Review*, *18*(3), 345–362.
Kozlov, V. (2000). *The Butcher of Rostov: The true story of Andrei Chikatilo*. HarperCollins.
Lev, A. (1998). *Chikatilo: The monstrous history of Russia's most notorious serial killer*. St. Martin's Press.
Smith, R. (2014). Psychopathic behavior and serial murder: An analysis. *Psychological Review*, *121*(1), 35–52.

8

CASE STUDY ON TED KACZYNSKI

Introduction

Theodore John Kaczynski also known as "Unabomber" was an American domestic terrorist, anarchist, and mathematics prodigy from Harvard University. He is best known for a campaign of letter bombs he sent as the "Unabomber," which stands for "University and Airline Bomber," over a 20-year period, resulting in three fatalities. Kaczynski taught at the University of California at Berkeley before he retreated to a primitive lifestyle in the woods. He moved to a remote cabin without electricity or running water near Montana, where he lived as a recluse while learning survival skills to become self-sufficient. He began his bombings in 1978 during his reclusive period. He wrote frequent letters to different media firms such as the *Washington Post* and the *New York Times*, with a final manifesto titled Industrial Society and Its Future (FBI, 1996).

Between 1978 and 1995, Kaczynski engaged in mailing or hand-delivering a series of bombs that cumulatively killed three people and injured 23. The bombings were primarily aimed at universities and airline officials. In 1995, Kaczynski released a 35,000-word manifesto titled Industrial Society and Its Future. In 1980, chief agent John Douglas, working with the Behavioral Sciences Unit, issued the psychological profile of the bomber. It described the individual as a man with above-average intelligence and links to academia. Using linguistic analysis, FBI agents arrested Kaczynski in 1996, at his cabin, in an unkempt state. He was indicted. After the rejection of a defense based on anti-technology views, Kaczynski tried to commit suicide by hanging on January 9th (FBI, 1996).

DOI: 10.4324/9781003602927-10

Background

Ted Kaczynski was born on May 22, 1942, in Chicago, Illinois, the oldest child of a Polish-American couple. During his fourth grade, he scored an IQ at 167. Thus, he skipped the sixth grade. All his neighbors considered him to be "strictly a loner..." and "a genius." In his school, he was regarded as an "outsider" by his classmates, calling him "a walking brain" and "smartest kid in class. He excelled at his academics with intense interest in Math, and skipped the eleventh grade, therefore graduating college at age 15. He entered Harvard University at age 16 on a scholarship" (Chase, 2003).

He was considered a "genius," as he earned his BA in Mathematics in 1962. In 1967, Kaczynski became the youngest assistant professor of mathematics in the history of University of California, Berkeley. He resigned in 1969 without any explanation. After 2 years, he moved to a remote cabin in Montana woods. He lived a simple life with little money and without electricity or running water, working odd jobs and receiving meager financial support from his family. He became averse to the use of modern technology and lived a life as a recluse (Chase, 2003).

Murray's Psychological study (1962): Kaczynski participated in a study by Henry Murray which was described as a "purposely brutalizing psychological experiment." The subjects were made to write essays detailing their personal beliefs and aspirations. Following this, the material was handed over to an attorney, who would then confront and belittle the subject, making personal attacks, and using their content. During the session, electrodes monitored the subject's physiological reactions. These encounters were filmed, and the subject's reaction was later played back to them multiple times. The experiment went on for a period of 3 years, with verbal abuse and humiliation happening each week; Kaczynski spent 200 hours as part of the study (Chase, 2019).

Developing from Ted's infancy, several biological inferences are prominent in his unhealthy development. As an infant, he had an allergic reaction to medication and had to spend time in isolation recovering. Report states that he had a noticeable change in personality after being hospitalized. This sense of isolation could have resulted in a disturbed attachment style, and led to changes in the child's biological functioning as well. The perceived threat or provocation leads to lower levels of serotonin, which leads to aggressive behavior. The interaction between low serotonin and high testosterone levels can have a significant effect on the neural mechanisms involved in aggression (Birger et al., 2003). The association is bidirectional, as low levels of serotonin can also heighten one's sensitivity or reactivity to cues of hostility or provocation (Krämer, Riba, Richter, & Munte, 2011). Norepinephrine and dopamine may also have affected the arousal and environmental sensitivity, leading to negative behavioral activation and goal-directed behavior in adulthood.

His high IQ of 167 made him skip grade six; the cognitive abilities involving activities of the frontal lobe and the prefrontal cortex in particular could be the primary neuroanatomical sites. The mixture of high cognitive functioning added with dysregulated neurochemical factors from infancy or predisposition could be one possible hypothesis for Kaczynski's antisocial behavior (Calkins & Keane, 2009).

A genetic predisposition toward narcissism is observed, Ted's background and education being contributive factors (Gupta, 2018). This would also account for the lack of empathy, as individuals with narcissistic personality shows abnormalities in the insular cortex. As observed in his manifesto, Kaczynski showcased a high regard for his beliefs and self. The disturbing aspect of narcissism, known as malignant narcissism, comes in when grandiosity is built around aggression and the destructive aspects of the self become idealized (Weigert, 1967). The significant neurocircuitry associated with empathy is the limbic system, primarily the hypo-activity in the amygdala, the ventromedial, and the orbitofrontal cortex, which is observed in antisocial behavioral traits (Anderson & Kiehl, 2014).

The psychological study by Murray, which induced extreme stress, could have increased agonistic behaviors (Haller, Harold, Sandi, & Neumann, 2014). Considering Kaczynski was only 16 when he joined Harvard, he might have been going through his peri-pubertal period, and the interaction between stress and hormonal changes could have resulted in pathological aggression, and a profound impact on his emotionality. With regard to emotionality, due to his reserved and limited social interaction, social isolation stress would have been present. This results in endocrinological changes such as activating the hypothalamic-pituitary axis (HPA) and other hormonal changes. Peri-pubertal stress leads to lowered anxiety-like behavior, increased risk-taking, and reduced sociability in adulthood (Haller et al., 2014).

Puberty is a period of special sensitivity for programming of aggressive and emotional behaviors due to stress, and this seems to be also the critical negative period in Ted's life. The prominent risk factors associated with aggressive and antisocial behavior are characteristics of the child and the characteristics of different social contexts. Social contexts such as family dysfunction, neighborhood dysfunction, and peer rejection are the important ones (Dodge et al., 2003). While all three were present during Kaczynski's developing phase, Kaczynski's personality traits such as quiet, reserve and intelligence, interacted with these social contexts.

When children skip a grade in an effort to keep their mind intellectually challenged, the potential accompanying social issues are overlooked. Some children are able to adapt, and some are not. Clearly, Kaczynski had the latter consequence; added to his reserved character; this would have made him feel more isolated. Research evidence states that social adjustment difficulties are generally found in children with IQ over 165, and more than two-thirds of them are defined as solitary or "poor mixers" (Burks, Jensen, & Terman, 1930).

With regard to neighborhood and communal dysfunction, Kaczynski's family shifted to a suburban community in Chicago to surround him with a higher class of friends. This move had an adverse effect, as the community soon became a racially mixed community, therefore isolated and discriminated against. The family got isolated due to the race wars, and children who were Ted's playmates got dispersed into different schools, which resulted in a home and school environment where he didn't know anyone. The social isolation became more prominent, as in school he mingled with older kids due to his intellectual advancement. The only appropriate age group was not there (Lieberman, 2000).

Another important social role which affected Kaczynski's negative attitudes was the teaching environment. The peer influence on antisocial behavior is found to be significantly greater then pro-social behavior, and individuals with less peer influence tend to have increased teacher influence. In correspondence with this finding, when Kaczynski's faculty members presented the children with inappropriate college textbook material, with ideas and worldviews unfamiliar to them, unlike the rest, Ted's drive to learn more got him engrossed in the material. Therefore, while his classmates were engaged in recreational activities such as smoking, drinking and such, Kaczynski isolated himself further by spending time alone reading. It's quintessential to look at how Kaczynski's education partly groomed him for his life as a terrorist. He became an "alienated intellectual" due to social mismatches such as early admission to Harvard, shifting communities for better education, and grouping him with intelligent freshmen at university. He was highly influenced by Harvard's approach toward scientific research, and disregarding human experience in goal attainment, which also arose as he was the victim of Murray's torturous study (Chase, 2019).

Criminal Behavior

Kaczynski's bombing campaign lasted nearly two decades, resulting in 3 deaths and 23 injuries. His carefully crafted explosive devices were sent through the mail or hand-delivered, targeting universities, airlines, and individuals associated with technological advancement. The name Unabomber was derived from the "University and airline bombing" or UNABOM task force that was set up to find the culprit behind the bombing series. The meticulous planning and execution of his attacks allowed him to evade capture for an extended period. His ability to remain elusive was a testament to his detailed operational planning and the challenges faced by law enforcement in tracking down the perpetrator (FBI, 1996; Wessler, 2001).

The first victim of Kaczynski was a material engineering professor at the University of Illinois, Buckley Crist, who received a package with his address as the return address. He called the campus security as he was sure he had not sent the package. The bomb detonated when campus security opened the package, injuring him. The next bomb, enclosed in a cigarette box, detonated and injured a graduate student in Northwestern University. He then proceeded to bomb an airplane, which only set off smoke and did not kill anyone because of a faulty timer. He then proceeded to mail the bomb to the US Airlines President, Percy Woods, who was injured. The next series of bombings were all targeted toward universities and computer stores. His last two victims were both industrialists, whom Kaczynski viewed as a threat to the environment and who were killed on their opening the bombs (FBI, 1996).

Kaczynski's bombs were sophisticated and designed out of scrap materials. The letters FC which stood for Freedom Club were etched onto the bombs. Kaczynski took care to wipe off his fingerprints on the bomb and also planted fingerprints on the bomb to mislead the investigators. In 1995, Kaczynski sent his manifesto to the FBI, demanding it be published by a major publisher. He mainly addressed technological revolution as curbing human freedom, demanding for an anti-leftist revolution (FBI, 1996).

Psychological Profile

Kaczynski's psychological profile suggests traits consistent with paranoid schizophrenia and a severe personality disorder. His writings and behavior indicate a profound paranoia and a delusional belief system, marked by an intense distrust of modern society and technology. The combination of his isolation, intellectual superiority, and extreme ideological beliefs contributed to his psychological deterioration and subsequent criminal behavior (Hickey, 2016; Lieberman, 2000).

Ted Kaczynski, known as the "Unabomber," is one of the most infamous domestic terrorists in the US, responsible for a nearly two-decade-long bombing campaign that targeted people and institutions he viewed as emblematic of modern technology and industrial society. His psychological profile offers a complex case study of a man with extraordinary intelligence and deep-seated resentment toward societal systems, who gradually detached from society and developed a violent anti-technology ideology. Kaczynski was born in 1942; his early years, his unique intellectual abilities, and his ideological transformation played key roles in his eventual turn toward extremism (Chase, 2003).

Kaczynski was born in Chicago and raised in a relatively stable, working-class family, with both parents described as caring and supportive. From an early age, he displayed exceptional intelligence, scoring an IQ of 167 on testing, which enabled him to skip grades and enter Harvard University at just 16 (Chase, 2003). However, his intellectual prowess was accompanied by significant social challenges. Accounts from his early years indicate that he struggled with social integration, feeling alienated and misunderstood by his peers. He was described as shy, emotionally reserved, and largely solitary—traits that, while often associated with introversion, may have signaled early signs of social difficulties and an underlying sensitivity to rejection and perceived inadequacies.

Kaczynski's adolescence and young adulthood showed marked signs of alienation. As he progressed through school, his social isolation deepened. Classmates described him as "odd" and "eccentric," someone who kept to himself and rarely engaged in social activities (Lieberman, 2000). This isolation became a defining feature of his personality, as he found solace in intellectual pursuits rather than human relationships. His move to Harvard furthered this sense of alienation. Despite his intellectual capabilities, he did not form close bonds with others at the university, which may have deepened his feelings of separateness from society. His extreme introversion and inability to relate socially contributed to a growing sense of frustration with societal norms, laying the groundwork for later resentments.

Kaczynski's psychological development took a pivotal turn at Harvard, where he participated in a controversial psychological study led by psychologist Henry Murray (Chase, 2019). This study, which some argue may have exacerbated Kaczynski's mental health struggles, involved intensive psychological stress tests designed to break down participants' egos by exposing them to intense interrogation and humiliation. Murray's study has been likened to a form of psychological torture, with subjects subjected to intense scrutiny, personal questioning, and emotional stressors intended to challenge their belief systems.

While it is difficult to assess the precise impact of the study, it is likely that the intense psychological pressures Kaczynski endured contributed to his growing distrust of authority figures and scientific institutions. This experience is often considered a catalyst for his eventual rejection of modern society and technology, planting seeds of resentment that he would later develop into a full-fledged ideology. Some psychologists have suggested that this experience may have exacerbated latent mental health issues, possibly triggering paranoid tendencies or contributing to a gradual erosion of his capacity for empathy and social trust.

After graduating from Harvard, Kaczynski completed his PhD in mathematics at the University of Michigan and briefly held an academic position at the University of California, Berkeley. However, his academic career was short-lived; in 1969, he resigned from his position, moving to a remote cabin in Montana where he would live in isolation for many years (Chase, 2019). This decision marked a profound shift in his life—one where his intellectual pursuits would turn toward examining and rejecting the very society that had once celebrated his intellect. Kaczynski's writings reveal a man deeply troubled by the effects of modern technology and industrialization, which he believed eroded human freedom and autonomy. His manifesto, *Industrial Society and Its Future*, argued that technological progress inevitably leads to the suppression of individual autonomy and the destruction of the natural environment (FBI, 1996). This belief became the core of his ideology, which he used to justify violent attacks against those he perceived as "agents" of technological enslavement.

Kaczynski's psychological profile is marked by signs of paranoid and obsessive thinking. He believed that technology posed an existential threat to human freedom and saw himself as a prophetic figure uniquely capable of understanding and resisting this threat. Psychologists who have studied his case suggest that he exhibited signs of schizoid personality disorder, which includes detachment from social relationships and a restricted range of emotional expression. However, Kaczynski's mental health diagnosis remains ambiguous, with some experts arguing that his extreme introversion and ideological rigidity might not fully qualify as a diagnosable mental illness. Instead, his paranoia, obsession with control, and emotional detachment contributed to a deeply ingrained worldview that became increasingly rigid and disconnected from reality. Kaczynski's self-imposed isolation in Montana served to deepen his ideological convictions. Living alone in a remote cabin, he lacked the social connections that might have challenged or softened his views. His isolation likely intensified his feelings of resentment and paranoia, as he had little opportunity for social feedback or alternative perspectives. Gradually, he began to see violence as a legitimate means of achieving his anti-technological goals, believing that targeted attacks could inspire a societal movement against industrial society.

His turn toward violence reflects an underlying desire for control, a theme that appears consistently throughout his life. By mailing bombs to individuals and institutions he deemed complicit in technological oppression, he believed he could exert a form of influence over society. The meticulous planning, careful construction of bombs, and selection of targets indicate obsessive tendencies and a need for precision and control, which further hint at possible obsessive-compulsive features. Kaczynski's actions were widely condemned as morally reprehensible, yet his case raises complex questions about the relationship between mental health and ideology-driven violence. His writings and behavior suggest a man deeply troubled by his inability to reconcile his intellectual ideals with societal realities. While some elements of his behavior align with psychopathological symptoms, it remains difficult to distinguish between his ideology and any potential mental illness. For instance, while paranoia can be symptomatic of a mental disorder, it can also be a component of ideological extremism when fueled by a rigid belief system and social isolation.

Ted Kaczynski's psychological profile is a study in the intersection of extraordinary intellect, social alienation, and ideological rigidity. His isolation, mistrust of society, and rejection of human relationships contributed to the development of an extremist worldview that justified violence as a means to an ideological end. Kaczynski's case is illustrative of how profound social isolation and unchecked ideological beliefs can lead to violent outcomes. He was a person of rare intellectual talent but with a personality shaped by withdrawal, alienation, and an extreme need for control. His story underscores the risks associated with untreated psychological issues in individuals whose intellect and beliefs may provide them with a sense of justification for harming others. In his later years, Kaczynski remained unrepentant, adhering to the same rigid worldview that drove his violent campaign—a testament to the enduring power of unchallenged beliefs and the dangerous potential of ideologically motivated violence.

Possible Treatment

Addressing Kaczynski's mental health issues would have been challenging due to his severe paranoid schizophrenia and entrenched personality disorder. Antipsychotic medications and cognitive-behavioral therapy (CBT) could have potentially managed his delusional thoughts and paranoia. However, Kaczynski's profound mistrust of mental health professionals and societal institutions would have likely posed significant obstacles to effective treatment. His deep-seated beliefs and isolation further complicated any therapeutic intervention (Hickey, 2016; Barlow & Durand, 2014).

Captivation and Trial

The Unabom task force was established as early as 1979, post the airline bombings, comprising the FBI, the ATF, and the US Postal services. The task force received a profile of the Unabomber from the Behavioral Science Unit of the FBI in 1980. Kaczynski was apprehended in 1996 after his brother recognized his writing style in the manifesto published by the media and alerted authorities. During his trial, Kaczynski attempted to represent himself but eventually pled guilty to avoid the death penalty. He was sentenced to life imprisonment without the possibility of parole, a verdict reflecting both the severity of his crimes and the complexity of his psychological condition (FBI, 1996; Tise, 1997).

Conclusion

The Unabomber case provides a stark illustration of the intersection between severe mental illness and criminal behavior. Analyzing Kaczynski's psychological profile offers valuable insights into the factors driving individuals to commit acts of terrorism and underscores the critical need for early intervention and effective treatment for severe mental disorders.

References

Anderson, N. E., & Kiehl, K. A. (2014). Psychopathy: Developmental perspectives and their implications for treatment. *Restorative Neurology and Neuroscience*, *32*(1), 103–117. https://doi.org/10.3233/rnn-139001

Barlow, D. H., & Durand, V. M. (2014). *Abnormal psychology: An integrative approach* (7th ed.). Cengage Learning.

Birger, M., Swartz, M., Cohen, D., Alesh, Y. A., Grishpan, C., & Kotelr, M. (2003). Aggression: The testosterone-serotonin link. *Israel Medical Association Journal*, *5*(9), 653–658.

Burks, B. S., Jensen, D. W., & Terman, L. M. (1930). *Genetic studies of genius*. III. *The promise of youth*. Stanford University Press.

Calkins, S. D., & Keane, S. P. (2009). Developmental origins of early antisocial behavior. *Development and Psychopathology*, *21*(4), 1095–1109. https://doi.org/10.1017/s095457940999006x

Chase, A. (2003). *A mind for murder: The education of the Unabomber and the origins of modern terrorism*. W. W. Norton & Company.

Chase, A. (2019, September 6). Harvard and the making of the Unabomber. *The Atlantic*. https://www.theatlantic.com/magazine/archive/2000/06/harvard-and-the-making-of-the-unabomber/378239/?single_page=true

Dodge, K. A., Lansford, J. E., Burks, V. S., Bates, J. E., Pettit, G. S., Fontaine, R., & Price, J. M. (2003). Peer rejection and social information-processing factors in the development of aggressive behavior problems in children. *Child Development*, *74*(2), 374–393.

FBI. (1996). *The Unabomber case*. Federal Bureau of Investigation.

Gupta, A. (2018). A psychological accounting of a modern Luddite: Ted Kaczynski AKA the Unabomber. *Psychology and Psychotherapy: Research Study*, *2*(1), 1–7.

Haller, J., Harold, G., Sandi, C., & Neumann, I. D. (2014). Effects of adverse early-life events on aggression and anti-social behaviours in animals and humans. *Journal of Neuroendocrinology*, *26*(10), 724–738.

Hickey, E. W. (2016). *Serial murderers and their victims* (7th ed.). Cengage Learning.

Krämer, U. M., Riba, J., Richter, S., & Münte, T. F. (2011). An fMRI study on the role of serotonin in reactive aggression. *PLoS One*, *6*(11), e27668.

Lieberman, A. (2000). The psychology of terrorism: An analysis of the Unabomber. *Psychological Perspectives*, *43*(3), 291–304.

Tise, J. (1997). The trial of Ted Kaczynski: Legal and psychological implications. *Harvard Law Review*, *110*(8), 2401–2420.

Weigert, E. (1967). Narcissism: Benign and malignant forms. *Crosscurrents in Psychiatry and Psychoanalysis*, 222–238.

Wessler, S. (2001). The Unabomber: The man, the myth, the case. *Law & Order*, *49*(5), 26–34.

9

CASE STUDY ON ANDREA YATES

Introduction

Andrea Yates' case represents a profoundly tragic and complex study in forensic psychology involving a mother's severe mental illness and the devastating murder of her five children. This chapter explores Yates' background, psychological profile, and the legal and forensic aspects of her case, providing insights into the intersection of severe mental illness and criminal behavior.

Background

Andrea Yates grew up in the Houston region. She was born on July 2, 1964. She seemed to be from a middle-class, middle-American family. Shortly before the murders, her father, passed away from Alzheimer's illness. Jutta Karin, her mother, was a housewife. As the youngest of five children, Yates was expected to excel in high school, and she did just that, becoming the swim team captain, a member of the National Honor Society, and the valedictorian of her graduating class in 1982. She continued to the University of Texas School of Nursing in Houston, where she graduated in 1986 after completing a 2-year pre-nursing program at the University of Houston. From 1986 to 1994, she was employed as a registered nurse at the University of Texas M.D. Anderson Cancer Center. However, Andrea's nursing career ceased entirely soon after her marriage to Rusty (Yates, 2002; Oates, 2004).

In 1989, while living in the same apartment complex in Houston, Andrea and Rusty first crossed paths. At the time, they were both 25. A summa cum laude graduate of Auburn University and "a popular jock" in high school, Rusty was working on computer systems for NASA. As Rusty would later

DOI: 10.4324/9781003602927-11

disclose, Andrea made the rather daring action of approaching him first in conversation. Rusty didn't find out until after Andrea's arrest that she hadn't dated until she was 23, that she was recovering from a breakup when they first met, and that her directness in reaching out to him was motivated by extreme loneliness and possibly melancholy. Over the course of the following few years, Andrea and Rusty got to know one another by "living together, reading the Bible, and praying" (Denno, 2017).

They had a modest and uncomplicated wedding ceremony on April 17, 1993. Perhaps as a result of Rusty's spiritual tutor, Michael Woroniecki, from whom "he had learned the faults of organized religion," it was also surprisingly non-denominational. The couple boldly declared to their wedding guests that they wanted as many children as nature would allow and that they would not use birth control. Their desire to have children was instantly granted. Andrea became pregnant with the first of her five children in just 3 months (McLellan, 2006).

Over the next 7 years, Andrea gave birth to five children and suffered one miscarriage, all the while plunging deeper into mental illness. Then on June 20, 2001, in less than an hour, Andrea drowned all of her children in the bathtub, one by one. Four months later, she was convicted of capital murder in Harris County, Texas, where she now serves a life sentence (McLellan, 2006).

Yates' struggle with severe mental illness, including schizophrenia, played a crucial role in her tragic actions. Her case highlights the challenges in diagnosing and treating severe psychological disorders and the profound impact these conditions can have on individuals and their families (Gordon, 2009).

Looking into Yates' family history of psychiatric illness, it can be seen that two of her siblings were diagnosed with depression, and one was diagnosed with bipolar disorder. After the birth of her fourth child, Yates showed signs of post-partum depression, which worsened over time. She was reported to have had delusional thoughts of Satan trying to kill her children. She attempted suicide twice within a span of 5 weeks in 1999. She was admitted to a psychiatric facility after each of the attempts. She was diagnosed with major depressive disorder with psychotic features. There was a relapse of post-partum depression with the birth of their fifth child in 2001. Yates' symptoms this time included suicidal thoughts, reduced appetite, and psychomotor activities, along with paranoid and referential delusions. She believed she was being monitored and even believed her mother-in-law was part of the surveillance. She also believed that her children would grow up to lead sinful lives and end up in hell after their deaths. She did not disclose any of these delusions to her family or psychiatrist for fear of them disclosing this information to the Devil (Resnick, 2007).

Criminal Behavior

In June 2001, Andrea Yates drowned her five children in the family's bathtub, an act driven by her delusional belief that she was saving them from eternal damnation. Her severe post-partum psychosis impaired her ability to distinguish between reality and delusion, leading to this horrific act (Krupnick, 2005; Swanson, Van Dorn, & Swartz, 2006). The crime shocked the public and sparked intense debate about the nature of mental illness and criminal responsibility.

Yates' behavior was characterized by a profound disconnect from reality, driven by her delusions and psychotic symptoms. Her actions highlighted the severe impact of untreated mental illness on behavior and judgment (Oates, 2004; Hall, 2006).

Yates believed that Satan was residing within her, which led to her and her children being tortured. She believed that she would free her children by killing them. Her arrest and execution post this will lead to Satan being killed with her. She thus drowned her five children, in no particular order. She then laid them down on the bed, called her husband and 911, informing them that she had killed her children (Resnick, 2007).

Psychological Profile

Andrea Yates, an American mother who drowned her five children in 2001, represents one of the most tragic cases in the history of forensic psychology. Her case illuminates the impact of severe mental illness, religious influences, and environmental stressors on behavior. Yates' actions shocked the nation and raised important questions about mental health, maternal responsibility, and the healthcare system's ability to provide effective treatment to individuals suffering from chronic psychiatric conditions. The following psychological profile of Yates explores the interplay of her psychological history, family dynamics, and environmental stressors that culminated in this tragedy.

Andrea Yates' descent into mental illness began shortly after the birth of her first child in 1994. She experienced post-partum depression, which went largely untreated. Her condition worsened with each subsequent birth, as she gave birth to five children between 1994 and 2000 in rapid succession. The stresses of raising a large family in a cramped, makeshift living space compounded her emotional strain, especially as Rusty believed in adhering to a traditional family structure where Andrea bore most of the childcare responsibilities (Resnick, 2007).

Yates' mental health deteriorated sharply after the birth of her fourth child, Luke, in 1999 (Resnick, 2007). She was hospitalized for severe depression, which progressed to psychosis. During her hospitalization, she attempted suicide twice and reported hearing voices telling her she was a "bad mother" and "deserved to be punished." She was diagnosed with post-partum psychosis—a rare but severe mental illness that affects a small percentage of women after childbirth and is associated with symptoms like delusions, hallucinations, paranoia, and irrational thinking. Doctors prescribed a range of medications, including antipsychotics, and advised against having more children, as further pregnancies could exacerbate her condition. However, Rusty and Andrea later chose to have a fifth child, Mary, in 2000, a decision that would prove devastating as her psychosis deepened (Resnick, 2007).

The influence of religious beliefs on Yates' psyche cannot be overstated. Andrea's exposure to fundamentalist Christian teachings, particularly those espoused by Michael Woroniecki, may have fueled her feelings of guilt, inadequacy, and fear of eternal damnation. Woroniecki's message, which emphasized that mothers bore the responsibility for their children's spiritual fate, likely intensified Andrea's belief that her children would be condemned if she could not "save" them. She became consumed by the notion that she was a failure as a mother and that her children were at risk of eternal suffering because of her shortcomings. These religious ideations became intertwined with her psychotic symptoms, forming a delusional system where she believed that the only way to protect her children was to end their lives.

Yates' delusions became progressively complex and irrational, underscoring the severity of her psychosis. She believed she was possessed by Satan and that her children would be damned because of her "evil" presence. In her mind, she was carrying out an act of mercy by taking their lives, freeing them from the sinful world and securing their place in heaven. This religiously driven delusional system not only motivated her actions but also provided a twisted justification for them, as she believed her actions were a necessary sacrifice for her children's salvation (Resnick, 2007).

Andrea Yates' mental health treatment was inconsistent and fraught with systemic issues. Despite her diagnosis of post-partum psychosis, her treatment was often interrupted or altered, and her condition remained unstable. At various points, she was prescribed Haldol, an antipsychotic medication, which seemed to stabilize her condition (Resnick, 2007). However, her psychiatrist discontinued the medication several weeks before the killings, despite her history of psychotic symptoms and suicide attempts. The removal of this stabilizing medication, combined with inadequate follow-up care, left Andrea vulnerable to a psychotic relapse.

Moreover, the family's decision to have a fifth child, against medical advice, further destabilized her mental health. Rusty's belief that Andrea could handle more children and his insistence on a traditional family structure placed her under immense pressure. He also ignored warnings from medical professionals to avoid leaving her alone with the children, even though she was exhibiting signs of severe mental distress. On the morning of the killings, Rusty left Andrea alone with the children for an hour, a window of time that she used to carry out the drownings (Resnick, 2007). These circumstances point to a tragic confluence of factors where family pressures, religious beliefs, and systemic gaps in mental health care intersected with deadly consequences.

On June 20, 2001, Andrea Yates drowned her five children one by one, beginning with her youngest, 6-month-old Mary, and ending with her oldest, 7-year-old Noah (Resnick, 2007). This act was carried out in a manner that suggests profound detachment from reality, as well as a total lack of rational decision-making capacity. Psychologists and psychiatrists who later evaluated Yates agreed that she was experiencing a psychotic episode at the time, marked by delusions and command hallucinations. In her mind, the act was a selfless sacrifice—an attempt to save her children from eternal damnation.

Andrea's psychological state during the murders was one of extreme dissociation and psychosis. She likely believed, at that moment, that she was carrying out a divine mandate. Her actions were not driven by malice or anger but rather by a warped sense of love and duty, a tragic misinterpretation of maternal responsibility influenced by her delusions and religious fervor.

The case of Andrea Yates highlights the tragic consequences of untreated and poorly managed severe mental illness, especially post-partum psychosis. Her descent into psychosis was marked by delusions, hallucinations, and profound religious guilt that fed her belief that her children were in danger of eternal damnation. Andrea's actions were the culmination of an array of factors: religious ideation, a history of mental illness, systemic failures in her psychiatric treatment, and the pressures of a rigid family structure.

Yates' case underscores the need for improved mental health services, especially for women suffering from post-partum psychosis, a rare but life-threatening condition. It also highlights the dangers of untreated delusional thinking and the critical importance of a supportive, understanding environment for those experiencing severe mental illness. While her actions were horrific, understanding the mental state that led her to such a tragic decision helps us empathize with the devastating effects that untreated mental illness can have on individuals and families.

Possible Treatment

Effective treatment for Yates' severe mental illness would have required a comprehensive approach, including psychiatric medication and intensive therapy. Antipsychotic medications and psychotherapy could potentially help manage symptoms of psychosis and schizophrenia, although treatment efficacy is highly individualized (Yates, 2002; Barlow & Durand, 2014). Early intervention and ongoing mental health support are critical for individuals with severe psychological disorders to prevent relapse and manage symptoms effectively (Harrison, 2007).

Captivation and Trial

Andrea Yates' trial focused on her mental state at the time of the murders. The defense argued that she was not criminally responsible due to her severe mental illness. Initially convicted of capital murder in 2002, her conviction was later overturned on appeal due to issues with expert testimony and the presentation of evidence. In a subsequent trial, Yates was found guilty but sentenced to life imprisonment, reflecting the court's consideration of her mental health in the context of criminal responsibility (Krupnick, 2005; Harrison, 2007). The forensic psychiatrists who appeared for the defense diagnosed Yates with schizoaffective disorder, and the psychiatrist who appeared for prosecution conferred with the finding that Yates had severe mental health disorder (Resnick, 2007).

To those closest to Andrea, this self-blaming reaction came as no surprise. They could testify that Andrea had been tormented by bouts of mental illness, and, in fact, both the prosecution and defense agreed that she was mentally ill. Andrea's life was also distinguished by religious obsession and steadfast devotion to tales of sin and Scripture, a "repent-or-burn zeal" that led her to believe she was a bad mother with ruined offspring. According to Andrea, she killed her children to save them from Satan and her own evil maternal influences, delusions that did little to help Andrea's defense because they fueled her own desire for punishment. Public opinion on the Yates killings helps explain some of the more contradictory themes in the case.

On the one hand, the public had much sympathy for Andrea and the life that she led. Yet, her composed behavior on the day she killed her children stirred a strong retributive response. Many were unable to comprehend such violence except by declaring it intentional and evil. According to this view, it could be said that Andrea was supremely sane—her acts rational and premeditated despite her unquestioned history of post-partum psychosis. Andrea propelled this account, spurring the public, her "jury," to see her as the Satanic mother she believed herself to be (McLellan, 2006).

Conclusion

The case of Andrea Yates underscores the complexities of mental illness and criminal responsibility. Her tragic actions and the legal proceedings highlight the challenges of balancing justice with understanding mental health issues. This case serves as a critical example of the need for effective mental health treatment and support, particularly for individuals experiencing severe psychological disorders.

References

Barlow, D. H., & Durand, V. M. (2014). *Abnormal psychology: An integrative approach* (7th ed.). Cengage Learning.

Denno, D. W. (2017). Andrea Yates: A continuing story about insanity. In *The insanity defense: Multidisciplinary views on its history, trends, and controversies* edited by Mark D. White (pp. 367–416). Praeger.

Gordon, M. (2009). Mental illness and criminal responsibility: The Andrea Yates case. *Journal of Forensic Sciences*, *54*(2), 287–295.

Hall, R. (2006). Postpartum psychosis: A comprehensive review. *Psychiatric Clinics of North America*, *29*(1), 55–71.

Harrison, R. (2007). Early intervention in severe mental illness: A review. *Clinical Psychology Review*, *27*(5), 486–496.

Krupnick, M. (2005). *The Andrea Yates case: A study in mental illness*. Random House.

McLellan, F. (2006). Mental health and justice: the case of Andrea Yates. *The Lancet*, *368*(9551), 1951–1954. https://doi.org/10.1016/s0140-6736(06)69789-4

Oates, M. (2004). Understanding postpartum psychosis: A case study. *Archives of Women's Mental Health*, *7*(2), 121–128.

Resnick, P. J. (2007). The Andrea Yates case: Insanity on trial. *Cleveland State Law Review*, *55*(2), 147. https://engagedscholarship.csuohio.edu/cgi/viewcontent.cgi?article=1174&context=clevstlrev

Swanson, J. W., Van Dorn, R. A., & Swartz, M. S. (2006). The relationship between mental illness and violence: Findings from the MacArthur Violence Risk Assessment Study. *Journal of Clinical Psychiatry*, *67*(7), 905–912.

Yates, A. (2002). *Andrea Yates: The story of a mother's madness*. HarperCollins.

PART III

High-Profile Criminal Minds

10

CASE STUDY OF YORKSHIRE RIPPER

Introduction

Peter Sutcliffe, infamously known as the Yorkshire Ripper, is one of the most notorious serial killers in British history. Between 1975 and 1980, Sutcliffe was responsible for the brutal murders of 13 women, leaving a trail of terror and fear across Yorkshire (Steel, n.d.). This chapter explores Sutcliffe's psychological profile, the details of his criminal behavior, and the forensic and investigative techniques used to capture him.

Background

Peter William Sutcliffe was born on June 2, 1946, into a working-class family in Bingley, West Riding, of Yorkshire. His parents, John William Sutcliffe (1922–2004) and Kathleen Frances Coonan (1919–1978) of Connemara, had different religious backgrounds: Kathleen was a Roman Catholic, while John was active in the Anglican church choir at St. Wilfred's. The children were raised Catholic, with Sutcliffe briefly serving as an altar boy. Born prematurely, he spent 2 weeks in the hospital, and his mother, a victim of domestic violence, likely endured significant emotional stress during her pregnancy (Steel, n.d.).

John Sutcliffe, a heavy drinker, was known to be abusive, once striking Sutcliffe on the head with a beer glass, for sitting in his chair during a Christmas gathering. He held strong animosity toward his own mother, describing her as "a bitch," and refrained from speaking about her further. He frequently demeaned Sutcliffe, referring to him as "a wimp" and "a mummy's boy." Kathleen, in contrast, showed Sutcliffe considerable affection, leading

DOI: 10.4324/9781003602927-13

him to view her as "perfect." John would also discipline his children with a belt, and Sutcliffe's siblings later depicted their father as "a monster," noting that his presence would darken the household atmosphere due to his preoccupations with sports, choir, and womanizing (Keppel & Birnes, 2003).

In 1970, John Sutcliffe publicly humiliated Kathleen by pretending to be her lover to stage an encounter at a hotel, where he revealed evidence of her supposed infidelity in front of their children. During his late teenage years, Sutcliffe developed an increasing interest in voyeurism, often observing sex workers and their clients. Known as a loner, he left school at 15 and held various unskilled jobs, including two periods as a gravedigger at Bingley Cemetery, where he developed a dark sense of humor. Colleagues noted his unusual enthusiasm for the job, even volunteering for additional duties involving corpse handling. Between 1971 and 1973, Sutcliffe worked on a packaging line at Baird Television but left after being asked to take on a sales role (Jones, 2018).

Sutcliffe then took a night-shift position at Anderton International's Britannia Works in April 1973. After opting for redundancy in February 1975, he used part of his severance to train as a heavy goods vehicle (HGV) driver. However, he was dismissed from a subsequent job in March 1976 for stealing used tires. Unemployed for several months, he later found employment as an HGV driver for T. & W. H. Clark Holdings Ltd. in Bradford. Reports indicate that Sutcliffe may have hired sex workers during this period, and it is speculated that he once lost money to a sex worker and her accomplice. While some accounts do not confirm his use of their services, it is clear that he developed an intense fixation on observing them in Leeds and Bradford (Burn, 1993).

Sutcliffe met Sonia Szurma, then 16, whose family were refugees from Czechoslovakia, on February 14, 1967, in a pub within Bradford's red-light district. They married on August 10, 1974. Sonia, who was studying to become a teacher, was later diagnosed with paranoid schizophrenia. According to writer Gordon Burn, their relationship was marked by Sonia's dominance, with her sometimes reprimanding Sutcliffe "like a naughty schoolboy" and needing physical restraint during unprovoked outbursts of rage (Burn, 1993).

Journalist Barbara Jones, who interviewed Sonia extensively, found her to be "the most irritating, strangest and coldest person I've ever met." Sonia experienced multiple miscarriages and was eventually informed that she would not be able to have children. She later returned to her teaching course and briefly had an affair with an ice-cream vendor. In 1977, after completing her training and starting her teaching career, she and Sutcliffe used her earnings to purchase a home at 6 Garden Lane in Heaton, where they resided at the time of Sutcliffe's arrest (Burn, 1993).

Criminal Behavior

Sutcliffe's modus operandi involved luring his victims to isolated locations, where he would violently attack them, often using a hammer and a screwdriver. His killing spree was characterized by a methodical approach, as he carefully selected his victims and executed his attacks with disturbing consistency. Sutcliffe's violence was not limited to murder; he also inflicted severe injuries and psychological trauma on his survivors (Benton, 1985; Hall, 1998).

The Yorkshire Ripper's behavior exhibited several key characteristics of organized serial killers. He demonstrated a clear pattern in his selection of victims, often targeting those he deemed "socially unacceptable." His attempts to evade capture included changing his appearance and using various aliases, but his eventual arrest was facilitated by a combination of forensic evidence and public information (Sutcliffe, 1981; Williams, 1995).

Sutcliff's first reported assault was of a prostitute, whom he hit with a stone. She did not press charges against him. His next three victims were struck on their head and had their abdomen or back slashed. He was not able to kill them as he was interrupted by passersby. The first murder victim of Sutcliff was Wilma Mary McCann, whom he bludgeoned to death with a hammer. In his initial days, he mostly killed prostitutes and many of them were mutilated. This earned him the name of Yorkshire Ripper, drawing a parallel to the infamous serial killer of the late 1800s, Jack the Ripper.

Psychological Profile

Peter Sutcliffe, also known as the "Yorkshire Ripper," terrorized the north of England from 1975 to 1980, murdering at least 13 women and attacking several others (Steel, n.d.). His psychological profile provides a troubling window into the mind of a violent offender whose motivations, personality, and social history blend complex elements of psychopathy, mental illness, and cultural influences. Sutcliffe's case has been widely studied by forensic psychologists and criminologists seeking to understand the interplay of psychological disorders, life experiences, and personality traits in serial offenders.

Peter Sutcliffe was born in 1946 in Bingley, West Yorkshire, to a working-class family. He was one of six children in a household marked by tension, conflict, and, by some accounts, abusive behavior from his father (Keppel & Birnes, 2003). Growing up, Sutcliffe displayed signs of shyness, introversion, and social isolation. As a child, he was described as timid, awkward, and sensitive, traits that set him apart from his more outgoing, boisterous siblings and may have contributed to his feelings of alienation and inferiority.

During adolescence, Sutcliffe continued to struggle socially, often described as a "loner" who had difficulty making friends. Classmates and acquaintances observed that he seemed uncomfortable around girls, possibly due to a sense of sexual inadequacy and insecurity. These feelings were exacerbated by his father's high expectations and attempts to toughen him up through activities he found distressing. Psychological experts have suggested that his relationships with women later in life were impacted by these early experiences, as they may have contributed to a deeply internalized resentment and hostility toward women, feelings that became key elements of his future crimes.

In his early 20s, Sutcliffe began experiencing what he later described as religious visions and hearing voices, often associating these experiences with a divine mission. By his own account, these voices instructed him to kill prostitutes as part of a "mission from God" to rid the world of sin. He would later claim that these delusions drove his actions, believing he was divinely sanctioned to enact violence against women. This aspect of his personality—whether genuine psychosis or manipulative delusion—adds a complex layer to his psychological profile.

The religious aspect of Sutcliffe's delusional thinking is intertwined with his upbringing in a Catholic environment, which may have contributed to feelings of guilt, shame, and confusion about sexual matters. Some psychologists argue that this religious fervor, combined with latent sexual frustration and resentment, fed into his developing psychosis, shaping his perception of women, particularly those he saw as morally "corrupt." Sutcliffe's religiously tinged delusions became a core part of his self-narrative, allowing him to justify his violent behavior as part of a mission.

Sutcliffe's crimes reflect classic features of psychopathy, including lack of empathy, manipulation, and impulsivity. While he did not exhibit the typical charm associated with some high-profile psychopaths, he displayed other markers of antisocial personality disorder, such as an absence of remorse and pleasure in the suffering of others. Forensic experts have noted that his attacks were often meticulously planned and executed with precision, suggesting a level of premeditated control typical of psychopathic personalities. His ability to conceal his crimes for years also indicates a capacity for deception and manipulation, as he managed to evade police suspicion despite numerous interactions with law enforcement.

Sutcliffe's behavior toward his wife, Sonia, whom he married in 1974, further exemplifies the traits of a psychopath. Despite engaging in brutal, predatory behavior toward other women, he maintained a seemingly stable and affectionate relationship with his wife, a duality that allowed him to sustain a veneer of normalcy while hiding his violent impulses. This compartmentalization—exhibiting care and normalcy in one sphere of life while committing horrific crimes in another—is characteristic of psychopathic individuals who can mimic normative behaviors without truly experiencing the emotions associated with them.

The transition from harboring violent fantasies to acting upon them is a critical phase in the life of a serial killer. Sutcliffe's first recorded attack occurred in 1969, when he struck a woman with a hammer but left her alive.

Over the years, he would commit at least 13 murders and 7 additional attempted murders, targeting primarily sex workers in the red-light districts of northern England. His choice of weapon—usually a hammer, followed by stabbing with a knife—demonstrates an inclination toward intimate, hands-on methods of killing, which indicates both an appetite for control and a sense of anger toward his victims. Sutcliffe's violence appears to have been sexually motivated, as his attacks involved targeting women in vulnerable situations, particularly those working in prostitution.

Throughout his killing spree, Sutcliffe exhibited signs of ritualistic behavior. He often selected victims from specific areas and exhibited certain methods of approach and attack, establishing a consistent modus operandi that was eventually noted by police. This pattern of behavior reflects a methodical approach to violence, where his fantasies and needs were ritualized and repeated, a common trait among serial offenders who derive psychological satisfaction from structured, controlled acts of violence.

When Sutcliffe was finally apprehended in 1981, he claimed that he was driven by voices commanding him to kill. This defense led to significant debate among forensic experts about whether he suffered from paranoid schizophrenia, as he claimed, or whether he was simulating symptoms to avoid a harsher sentence. Some psychiatrists concluded that he exhibited clear signs of schizophrenia, including delusions and hallucinations, which supported his narrative of divine instructions. Others argued that Sutcliffe's behavior aligned more closely with psychopathy and antisocial personality disorder, emphasizing his lack of empathy, manipulation, and calculated approach to his crimes.

Ultimately, Sutcliffe was diagnosed with paranoid schizophrenia, which led to his transfer from prison to a high-security psychiatric hospital. However, some experts remain skeptical of this diagnosis, pointing out that Sutcliffe's symptoms could be consistent with malingering, where a person fabricates or exaggerates mental illness for secondary gain. It is possible that he exploited the appearance of psychotic symptoms to avoid the consequences of his actions, although the persistence of these symptoms over time lends credibility to his claims of schizophrenia.

Several motivations appear to have fueled Sutcliffe's actions, including anger, sexual frustration, and a sense of power over his victims. His background, characterized by a troubled upbringing, religious guilt, and social isolation, combined with signs of possible mental illness, created fertile ground for the development of violent fantasies that he ultimately enacted. The cultural context of 1970s England, where sex workers were often marginalized and seen as easy targets, also played a role. Sutcliffe's view of women as morally inferior, combined with his religious delusions, may have further distorted his perception, fueling his hatred and justifying his actions in his own mind.

Peter Sutcliffe's psychological profile combines elements of psychopathy, mental illness, and environmental factors that ultimately led to his transformation into a violent serial offender. His early life was marked by social isolation, religious influences, and feelings of inadequacy that culminated in a warped perception of women and sexuality. His violent actions were both psychopathic and delusional in nature, marked by a consistent modus operandi and an evident pleasure in exerting power over his victims. Sutcliffe's case underscores the complex interplay between psychopathy, mental illness, and social influences, highlighting the multifaceted nature of serial offenders and the challenges they pose for the criminal justice and mental health systems.

Possible Treatment

Effective treatment for Sutcliffe's severe mental disturbances would have required a multifaceted approach, including psychiatric medication and intensive therapy. Antipsychotic medications and psychotherapy might help manage symptoms of delusional thinking and violent tendencies, although the efficacy of treatment is highly individualized. Given Sutcliffe's antisocial personality traits and sexual sadism, specialized interventions focusing on impulse control and empathy development would be essential. Continuous monitoring and support would be necessary to prevent potential relapses and manage ongoing psychological issues.

Captivation and Trial

Peter Sutcliffe was apprehended in January 1981 after an extensive investigation that led to his identification and arrest. Sutcliffe was driving with a prostitute in his car when he was arrested by the police, who noticed his false plates. His physical description matched some features as described by witnesses and he was held for questioning. Police also recovered a hammer, rope, and knife near the place he was arrested. Following a strip search and questioning, Sutcliffe admitted his crimes and claimed that he was getting rid of the filth by killing prostitutes. His capture was facilitated by a combination of forensic evidence and witness statements, which linked him to the crimes. During his trial, Sutcliffe pleaded guilty to the murders and was sentenced to life imprisonment (Benton, 1985; Hall, 1998).

Sutcliffe's trial was highly publicized and generated significant media attention. His defense team argued that he was suffering from a mental illness at the time of the murders, but the court largely rejected this claim. Sutcliffe was convicted of 13 murders and several assaults, and he was sentenced to life imprisonment without the possibility of parole (Taylor, 2002; Williams, 1995).

Conclusion

The Yorkshire Ripper case remains a seminal study in forensic psychology and criminal investigation. Peter Sutcliffe's crimes and subsequent capture provide valuable insights into the behavior of serial killers and the techniques used to apprehend them. The case underscores the importance of psychological profiling and forensic analysis in solving complex and high-profile criminal cases.

References

Benton, T. (1985). *The Yorkshire Ripper: The case of Peter Sutcliffe*. Macmillan.
Burn, G. (1993). *Somebody's husband, somebody's son: The Story of the Yorkshire Ripper*. Arrow.
Hall, T. (1998). *The Yorkshire Ripper: Peter Sutcliffe's killing spree*. Allen & Unwin.
Jones, S. (2018, September 18). Who is the Yorkshire Ripper Peter Sutcliffe? History of notorious killer. *The Mirror*. https://www.mirror.co.uk/news/uk-news/who-yorkshire-ripper-peter-sutcliffe-8616762
Keppel, R. D., & Birnes, W. J. (2003). *The psychology of serial killer investigations:* The Grisly Business Unit. Academic Press.
Steel, F. (n.d.). Peter Sutcliffe—A killer's mask. Crime Library. https://www.crimelibrary.org/serial_killers/predators/sutcliffe/mask_1.html
Sutcliffe, P. (1981). *Confessions of a killer*. Penguin Books.
Taylor, S. (2002). *The* Yorkshire Ripper*:* Peter Sutcliffe's crimes. Harcourt.
Williams, P. (1995). *The manhunt for the Yorkshire Ripper*. Bloomsbury.

11

CASE STUDY ON LUIS GARAVITO

Introduction

Luis Alfredo Garavito Cubillos was a Colombian homosexual pedophile sadist and serial killer who is also known as "The Beast," "Tribilin," or "The Monster of Genova." He was born on January 25, 1957, in Genova, Colombia, and was the eldest of seven children. He had a tough childhood and attended school for only a few years. It is speculated that his mother was a prostitute and his father was an alcoholic who abused his mother, siblings, and him. He was also forced by his father to watch while his mother engaged with her clients, and he also was sexually abused by these men. At the age of 8, he ran away from home and became a victim of sexual abuse by a pedophile. Additionally, he had a long history of alcohol and psychiatric illness (Jenkins, 2019).

In the 1990s he was convicted of murdering around 189 boys, and in 1999, he admitted to torture, rape, and murder of 138 children and teenagers aged between 8 and 16 years (Jenkins, 2019). According to a scientific report by Benecke (2002), he killed more than 200 children aged between 8 and 13 years of age from 1992 to 1999. He also had a stable modus operandi, which was targeting children of low economic status during daytime and luring them to isolated places and then tying the children up, then torturing and raping them, and then killing them (Benecke, 2002). He is also named "the world's worst serial killer" by the media and is at the top of the list in terms of confirmed victims. For all his crimes, he was sentenced to a total of 1853 years and 9 days of jail time, the longest sentence in Colombian history. Based on this case, the main aim of this chapter is to evaluate his criminal behavior based on the biopsychosocial model of criminal behaviors.

DOI: 10.4324/9781003602927-14

Background

Growing up in a low socio-economic status and facing a turbulent childhood, he lacked nurturing familial relationships. Both his parents were neglectful, and his family was dysfunctional. He was allowed to go to school only till the fifth grade, and even till that time, he was constantly bullied by his peers. His father only interacted with him for work-related matters and forbade him from having any relationships outside the family (Jenkins, 2019).

Research by Åslund et al. (2013) indicates that adolescent boys with the LL genotype (homozygous for the long allele) from low socio-economic backgrounds are at higher risk of delinquent behavior. With limited education and adverse living conditions, he eventually left home and had no stable role model to guide him in discerning right from wrong. Instead, he learned behaviors by modeling them in his immediate environment. As noted by Sigfusdottir, Farkas and Silver (2004), adolescents in conflict-ridden home environments often experience heightened anger, likely further impacting their development.

Numerous genetic theories have used twin studies to explore the potential hereditary basis of criminal behavior, revealing a correlation between genetics and such tendencies. While genetic predispositions may exist, environmental factors also significantly influence behavioral outcomes; it is the interaction of both that often contributes to criminal conduct (Chakraborty, Upreti, & Mishra, 2011). In this case, his father was notably abusive toward him, his mother, and his siblings, indicating a volatile environment that could have strengthened any inherent predispositions. Thus, his inherited tendencies, combined with exposure to violence and abuse, may have reinforced maladaptive beliefs and behaviors.

Garavito had claimed that a neighbor had molested him as a child. He became more withdrawn after this experience. He exhibited cruelty toward animals and behaved in a sexually inappropriate manner to his younger siblings (Jenkins, 2019). His experiences of childhood sexual abuse appear to have profoundly impacted his behavior. Research by Felson and Lane (2009) reveals that male offenders often reenact their own abusive experiences, particularly those involving sexual abuse, which may explain their subsequent actions. Such behavior aligns with social learning theory, which posits that children subjected to abuse are more likely to display similar abusive tendencies as adults. His own patterns of luring victims mirrored the approach used by his abusers, reinforcing this behavioral cycle.

As a teen, Garavito had attempted to sexually abuse young boys on multiple occasions. He was thrown out of his home and other residences for this reason. During this time, he had tried to hold on to a steady job, but his aggressive tendencies and drinking behavior got him fired. He resorted to working as a laborer and street vendor. His girlfriends and friends had noted that he was only aggressive when drinking (Jenkins, 2019).

His dependence on alcohol can be attributed to both biological and social influences. His father, reportedly an alcoholic, may have passed on a predisposition toward alcohol dependency. Mackie, Conrod, Rijsdijk and Eley (2011) found that genetic inheritance can influence individuals to consume alcohol, often to mitigate negative emotions or for social reasons. However, social and environmental factors frequently amplify such tendencies. The family environment, as Mackie et al. (2011) indicate, significantly affects adolescent drinking behavior. Other environmental risk factors like poor social skills, lack of parental guidance, and a history of abuse likely contributed to his alcohol dependence. It was documented that he was often under the influence of alcohol when committing crimes (Benecke, 2002), supporting research that links alcohol dependence with a higher likelihood of engaging in violent behavior (Heinz, Beck, Meyer-Lindenberg, Sterzer, & Heinz, 2011). Such aggression has neurobiological roots, arising from cognitive deficits related to alcohol consumption and social origins, including previous exposure to alcohol-related conflict resolution, social discrimination, and exclusion during childhood (Beck & Heinz, 2013). These environmental stressors, coupled with genetic variations in serotonin-related genes, may increase amygdala activity and impair prefrontal cortex function, leading to heightened aggression (Heinz et al., 2011). His exposure to his father's aggressive behavior while intoxicated may have set a behavioral precedent, perpetuating his own alcohol-related aggression through social learning. His alcohol use may also reflect ineffective coping mechanisms, particularly given his likely sensitivity to stress. Some individuals turn to alcohol to escape negative emotions, a trend noted by Mackie et al. (2011).

He exhibited traits indicative of antisocial personality disorder (ASPD), including disregard for others' rights, deceitfulness, manipulation for personal gain, irritability, aggressiveness, and a lack of remorse. These characteristics align with the Diagnostic and Statistical Manual of Mental Disorders criteria for antisocial personality (American Psychiatric Association, 2013). He had psychotic symptoms, was depressed, and had suicidal ideations. He consulted occasionally with psychiatrists and went to Alcoholics Anonymous meetings. Garavito was unable to hold onto steady jobs or relationships. He read about astrology and Satanism and admired Hitler (Jenkins, 2019). His behavior—deceiving, bribing, and manipulating individuals—illustrates these traits. As he frequently changed jobs and was transient, his lack of stability further underscores a disregard for conventional norms. According to Ostrosky and Ardila (2017), individuals with antisocial personality traits who engage in psychopathic behavior are particularly dangerous, as they are adept at feigning emotions and manipulating others for their benefit.

Criminal Behavior

Garavito's criminal activities, which occurred between 1992 and 1999, involved the abduction, torture, and murder of over 100 young boys. His modus operandi included luring victims with promises of money, food, or gifts, often targeting impoverished and vulnerable children from rural areas. He either posed as people of authority like priests and social workers or as disabled and homeless to cater to the sympathy of his victims. Once in his control, Garavito subjected them to extreme violence and sexual assault, frequently recording his crimes on video. He sexually abused his victims, killed them, and mutilated their remains (Martínez, 2007).

His methods demonstrated a high degree of premeditation and sadistic pleasure. He used various tactics to gain the trust of his victims before subjecting them to brutal and prolonged torture. Garavito's crimes were characterized by a disturbing level of ritualistic behavior, and he often chose isolated locations to carry out his murders (Bermúdez, 2010). This approach allowed him to avoid detection and maintain control over his victims (Garavito, 2001).

He had claimed that prior to killing his first victim, he had received instructions to kill from the Devil while he was playing on the Ouija board. He had been a serial child molester until this point. His first murder victim was Juan Carlos, whom he sexually assaulted and killed. Police noted that Carlos' genitals had been removed by his assailant. Garavito, in his subsequent murders, followed the same pattern, often removing the toes and fingers of the victims to make it look like ritual killings. The mutilations of his later victims escalated to the point where they were disemboweled alive and even decapitated. He also had reported victims in Ecuador, a country neighboring Colombia (Chan, 2019).

Psychological Profile

Luis Alfredo Garavito, known as "The Beast," is considered one of the most prolific serial killers in modern history, with his confirmed killings of over 138 young boys in Colombia during the 1990s, though the actual number may be significantly higher (Jenkins, 2019). His psychological profile reveals a chilling blend of sadism, psychopathy, and deeply ingrained personality disorders. The Garavito case raises crucial questions regarding the impact of childhood abuse, the development of psychopathic tendencies, and the challenges of identifying and rehabilitating such offenders in a society where resources for mental health intervention are limited.

Garavito was born in 1957 in Génova, Colombia, into a highly dysfunctional family marked by poverty, abuse, and neglect. He was the oldest of seven siblings and endured both physical and sexual abuse from his father and other male figures in his early years. Reports indicate that his father was authoritarian and frequently violent, beating Garavito severely and often humiliating him in front of others (Jenkins, 2019). This environment, rife with physical and emotional trauma, likely contributed to an early sense of powerlessness and insecurity.

Exposure to sexual abuse in childhood is a significant risk factor for later violent sexual behavior, and Garavito's repeated victimization seems to have left him with unresolved rage and a skewed understanding of interpersonal relationships. Trauma-induced feelings of anger, humiliation, and helplessness often become internalized, potentially leading to dissociation, distorted perceptions of control, and an association of violence with power. In Garavito's case, these formative experiences created a foundation of deep-seated resentment and detachment from empathy and emotional connection.

Garavito exhibits many characteristics associated with psychopathy. Psychopathy is characterized by a constellation of traits, including a lack of empathy, superficial charm, grandiosity, impulsivity, manipulativeness, and an inability to form genuine emotional connections with others. Throughout his life, Garavito demonstrated an absence of remorse for his actions, describing his crimes in clinical detail during confessions but showing no signs of guilt or empathy for his young victims. This lack of emotional engagement and empathy is a hallmark of psychopathy and is thought to arise from a combination of genetic predisposition and environmental influences like abuse and neglect.

Furthermore, Garavito's ability to deceive, charm, and manipulate people to achieve his goals is another characteristic common among psychopathic individuals. He was known to adopt various disguises and identities, including posing as a priest, monk, street vendor, and charity worker to lure boys into isolated areas. This strategic manipulation shows his proficiency in identifying others' vulnerabilities and exploiting them without hesitation.

Garavito's psychopathic tendencies may have been exacerbated by borderline personality features, particularly intense anger and self-image issues. Individuals with borderline personality disorder often experience unstable emotions and self-perceptions, as well as a pervasive fear of abandonment and impulsivity. His volatile emotional state, combined with a desire to regain control over feelings of inadequacy, could have driven his need to exercise power over his victims in a brutal and dehumanizing way.

A defining aspect of Garavito's psychological profile is his severe sexual sadism—a paraphilia characterized by deriving pleasure from inflicting pain, humiliation, or suffering on others. In his confessions, Garavito described how he would lure young boys, tie them up, and torture them before ultimately killing them, often using violent and degrading methods. For Garavito, inflicting pain was an essential part of his gratification. This sadistic drive is highly pathological and challenging to treat, as it involves reinforcing his sense of control and dominance over his victims.

Sexual sadism is often rooted in unresolved childhood trauma, where the perpetrator's earlier experiences of powerlessness and abuse are externalized onto vulnerable targets. In Garavito's case, his need to assert control over children—a group that mirrors his sense of vulnerability as a child—may have provided him with a twisted form of retribution. This gratification from causing suffering suggests a dissociative component to his psychology, where he effectively dehumanized his victims to avoid any empathy or guilt that might otherwise deter his actions.

Garavito's complex psychological makeup includes various paraphilias, including pedophilia and sadism, both of which were integral to his offending patterns. Pedophilia, the sexual attraction to prepubescent children, formed the basis of his victim selection, while sadism drove the brutal and prolonged suffering he inflicted on his victims. The combination of these two disorders creates a hazardous profile, as the drive to control, dominate, and inflict pain on vulnerable children becomes central to his motivations and self-perceived identity.

During his psychiatric evaluations, Garavito was also diagnosed with ASPD, a condition marked by disregard for social norms, impulsivity, lack of remorse, and the propensity to exploit others for personal gain. ASPD is common among serial offenders and may have contributed to his ability to carry out such heinous acts without conscience or ethical constraint. Although ASPD and psychopathy are related, the latter often involves additional traits like grandiosity, charm, and a more pronounced lack of emotional depth.

Garavito's modus operandi was calculated, systematic, and disturbingly efficient. He targeted vulnerable boys between the ages of 6 and 16, often from impoverished or displaced backgrounds, knowing that these children would not be immediately missed (Jenkins, 2019). His knowledge of the social environment allowed him to exploit gaps in the community and law enforcement. His approach of using disguises and luring techniques indicates a high level of premeditation, with each step of the abduction process carefully planned.

Typically, Garavito would gain the trust of his victims by offering them food, money, or work opportunities. Once isolated, he would subject them to hours of torture, mutilation, and eventually murder. The ritualistic aspect of his killings points to the compulsive nature of his violent fantasies, suggesting that he needed to fulfill a specific sequence of actions to derive satisfaction. This behavioral pattern is consistent with serial offenders who become addicted to the psychological and physical power exerted during their crimes.

When captured in 1999, Garavito provided detailed confessions of his crimes but exhibited little to no remorse. His statements were devoid of empathy as he recounted his actions in a detached, almost clinical manner. This detachment may reflect both psychopathy and the dissociative defenses that allowed him to commit his crimes without experiencing guilt. His remorse was likely minimal or nonexistent, as he viewed his victims as objects rather than human beings.

Luis Alfredo Garavito's psychological profile reveals a complex interplay of severe childhood trauma, psychopathic traits, sexual sadism, and paraphilias that culminated in his transformation into one of history's most notorious serial killers. His crimes were fueled by a deep-seated need to control, dominate, and inflict suffering on vulnerable children, behaviors driven by unresolved rage, psychopathic detachment, and sadistic fantasies.

Possible Treatment

Addressing Garavito's severe psychopathy and antisocial behavior would have posed significant challenges. Cognitive-behavioral therapy (CBT) and other conventional therapeutic approaches might have had limited effectiveness due to his deep-seated personality disorders and lack of remorse. Treatments would need to address both his psychopathic traits and his history of trauma (Hickey, 2016; González, 2005).

Effective management of such severe psychopathy typically requires long-term intervention, often involving a combination of psychotropic medications and structured therapeutic environments. However, given Garavito's severe and entrenched personality disorder, even these measures would likely have had limited success (Díaz, 2008; Rodríguez, 2012).

Captivation and Trial

Garavito was apprehended in 1999 after being identified by the authorities through forensic evidence and witness testimonies. His arrest followed a series of high-profile investigations and public appeals for information. Garavito's trial was a significant event in Colombia, revealing the full extent of his horrific crimes. He was convicted of multiple murders and sentenced to 22 years in prison, the maximum sentence permissible in Colombia at the time (Garavito, 2001; Martínez, 2007).

During his trial, Garavito's psychological profile and the details of his crimes were extensively examined, highlighting the complexities of his case and the challenges faced by law enforcement in capturing such a dangerous individual. The trial also brought attention to the need for improved mechanisms for tracking and managing sex offenders (Bermúdez, 2010; González, 2005).

Conclusion

Luis Garavito's case is a profound study of severe psychopathy and its impact on criminal behavior. His background, marked by severe abuse and trauma, combined with his psychopathic traits, drove him to commit heinous acts of violence. The case underscores the importance of understanding the complex interplay between psychological disorders and criminal behavior.

Garavito's crimes and subsequent capture provide critical insights into the behavior of serial killers and the investigative techniques used to apprehend them. The case highlights the need for effective mental health treatment and early intervention for individuals with severe personality disorders. It also emphasizes the importance of systemic improvements in monitoring and managing high-risk offenders to prevent similar tragedies (Hickey, 2016; Díaz, 2008).

References

American Psychiatric Association. (2013). *Diagnostic and statistical manual of mental disorders* (5th ed.). American Psychiatric Association.

Åslund, C., Comasco, E., Nordquist, N., Leppert, J., Oreland, L., & Nilsson, K. W. (2013). Self-reported family socioeconomic status, the 5-HTTLPR genotype, and delinquent behavior in a community-based adolescent population. *Aggressive Behavior*, *39*(1), 52–63.

Beck, A., & Heinz, A. (2013). Alcohol-related aggression—Social and neurobiological factors. *Deutsches Ärzteblatt International*, *110*(42), 711. https://doi.org/10.3238/arztebl.2013.0711.

Benecke, M. (2002). *Luis Alfredo Garavito Cubillos: Criminal and legal aspects of serial homicide with over 200 victims*. Archiv fur Kriminologie.

Bermúdez, L. (2010). *El monstruo de los Andes: La historia de Luis Garavito*. Editorial Planeta.

Chakraborty, D., Upreti, P. N., & Mishra, A. (2011). Genetic & environmental influences on criminal behaviour. *Calcutta Law Times*, *1*, 36.

Chan, H. C. (2019). A global casebook of sexual homicide. Springer *eBooks*. https://doi.org/10.1007/978-981-13-8859-0

Díaz, J. (2008). *Psicopatía y criminalidad: El caso de Luis Garavito*. Editorial Panamericana.

Felson, R. B., & Lane, K. J. (2009). Social learning, sexual and physical abuse, and adult crime. *Aggressive Behavior: Official Journal of the International Society for Research on Aggression*, *35*(6), 489–501. https://doi.org/10.1002/ab.20322

Garavito, L. A. (2001). *The Beast: The true story of Luis Garavito*. Random House.

González, M. (2005). *La mente del asesino: Un análisis del caso Garavito*. Editorial Norma.

Heinz, A. J., Beck, A., Meyer-Lindenberg, A., Sterzer, P., & Heinz, A. (2011). Cognitive and neurobiological mechanisms of alcohol-related aggression. *Nature Reviews Neuroscience*, *12*(7), 400. https://doi.org/10.1038/nrn3042

Hickey, E. W. (2016). *Serial murderers and their victims* (7th ed.). Cengage Learning.

Jenkins, J. (2019). Luis Garavito. Retrieved 8 December 2019, from https://www.britannica.com/biography/Luis-Garavito

Mackie, C. J., Conrod, P. J., Rijsdijk, F., & Eley, T. C. (2011). A systematic evaluation and validation of subtypes of adolescent alcohol use motives: Genetic and environmental contributions. *Alcoholism: Clinical and Experimental Research*, *35*(3), 420–430. https://doi.org/10.1111/j.1530-0277.2010.01359.x

Martínez, F. (2007). *Luis Garavito: El hombre detrás del horror*. Ediciones B.
Ostrosky, F., & Ardila, A. (Eds.) (2017). *Neuropsychology of criminal behavior*. Routledge.
Rodríguez, P. (2012). *Trastornos de la personalidad y criminalidad: El caso de Garavito*. Editorial Universitaria.
Sigfusdottir, I. D., Farkas, G., & Silver, E. (2004). The role of depressed mood and anger in the relationship between family conflict and delinquent behavior. *Journal of Youth and Adolescence*, *33*(6), 509–522.

12

CASE STUDY ON AILEEN WUORNOS

Introduction

Aileen Wuornos, a name synonymous with one of the most shocking cases of female serial killing in US history, committed a series of murders between 1989 and 1990 (Reynolds, 2016). This case study delves into Wuornos' psychological profile, exploring her traumatic background, the nature of her criminal behavior, and the underlying factors that led her down a path of violence and tragedy.

Background

Aileen Wuornos was born to her 14-year-old Finnish-American mother Diane Wuornos and 16-year-old father Leo Dale Pittman. Aileen's older brother Keith was born On March 14, 1955, and 2 months before Aileen was born, Diane filed for divorce. Wuornos never met her father, as he was incarcerated and convicted of sex crimes against children at the time of her birth. Her father Leo Dale was diagnosed with schizophrenia and committed suicide while in prison. Diane Pittman abandoned both her children who were later legally adopted by their maternal grandparents Lauri and Britta Wuornos. By the age of 11, Aileen Wuornos began engaging in sexual activities in school in exchange for cigarettes, drugs, and food, and even engaged in sexual activities with her own brother. Wuornos' parents and grandparents suffered from alcoholism. Throughout her childhood, she was sexually assaulted and raped by her grandfather. In 1970, at age 14, she became pregnant, having been raped by an accomplice of her grandfather, and gave birth to a boy who was put up for adoption. She soon dropped out of school around the same time

DOI: 10.4324/9781003602927-15

her grandmother died from liver failure. Her grandfather threw her out of the house, following which she supported herself by becoming a full-time prostitute at the age of 15 (Reynolds, 2016). At the age of 20, Aileen Wuornos met and married a rich 69-year-old businessman Lewis Fell. However, the marriage lasted only 9 weeks after which Fell filed for divorce on being assaulted by Wuornos. Following this, Wuornos was in and out of jail for charges of assault, armed robbery, and theft of a revolver, car, and ammunition. She soon engaged in a homosexual relationship with Tyria Moore, a hotel maid, and they lived together in a motel. Wuornos supported them with her earnings as a prostitute (Russell, 2002).

As previously mentioned, Aileen's biological father was a psychopath, diagnosed with schizophrenia, and a child sexual assaulter. There could be a possibility that she had inherited some of the psychopathic traits from her father, such as poor behavioral control, lack of remorse and empathy, which could have played an indirect role in causing her to commit crimes like murder. According to Blonigen et al. (2005), psychopathic traits can be inherited, making the offspring genetically predisposed and vulnerable. In the study conducted by Myers et al. (2005), Hare's Psychopathy Checklist Revised was utilized by the researchers to assess Aileen. The results generated from the checklist indicated that Aileen had a very high tendency of becoming a psychopath as she fulfilled a significant numbers of criteria in the checklist (with the total score of 30). It was reported that her mother, grandmother who died from liver failure, and grandfather were all alcoholics. Hence, there is a possibility that Aileen may have suffered from central nervous system damage or dysfunction due to prenatal alcohol exposure, which may have contributed to her aggressive personality and nature. As stated by Pinel (2014), prenatal alcohol exposure could cause neurological damage to a newborn, as well as disorders like lack of impulse control and difficulty to communicate. Being genetically predisposed as it is, Aileen Wuornos could also have had schizophrenia, paranoid schizophrenia to be more precise from her father, as toward the end, she experienced a complete psychological break.

In sum, by looking at the case of Aileen Wuornos from a biological perspective, it is possible that factors such as genetics and neurological dysfunction may have contributed to her criminal behavior.

Coming from a dysfunctional family and unhealthy environment, Wuornos developed a hot temper and aggressive behavior; she was more often than not rejected by peers and thus did not have many friends (Macleod, 2014). As stated by Bartol and Bartol (2014), studies have shown that children who are commonly rejected by peers are at high risk of developing antisocial and delinquent behavioral patterns. The statement is applicable to Aileen as she was involved in drug abuse, theft, and aggression toward peers as well as arson. Aileen Wuornos hated society and blamed society for making her the person she became. The Social Control Theory shows that

Wuornos' life experiences may have caused her to become a serial killer. Both her parents abandoned her; she was raped at a young age and kicked out of the only home she had as a teenager. These experiences caused her to lead a life of crime and earn a living as a prostitute. She dropped out of school at an early age, was alienated by her peers, and had few friends. School did not give her the social opportunities she was looking for in life (Reynolds, 2016). Thus, Wuornos was a product of her environment. Abandoned, abused, and alienated by society, Aileen Wuornos lived a life no human being would ever dream of wanting to live and this life eventually led to her serial murders.

Criminal Behavior

Wuornos' murder spree began in late 1989 and lasted until her arrest in January 1991. She was convicted of murdering seven men, whom she claimed were attempting to sexually assault her. Wuornos' modus operandi involved picking up men while working as a prostitute, shooting them, and then robbing them. Her actions reflected a blend of desperation and a survival instinct, driven by her traumatic experiences and unstable mental state (Foster, 2000; Hickey, 2016).

Wuornos began hitchhiking on highways, stopping middle-aged men and engaging in sexual activities with them. She would shoot them before they had sex, rob all of their money and belongings, and return to Moore. Aileen Wuornos was not an organized killer as she left her fingerprints all over the crime scenes. She killed seven men in the year 1990 (claimed to be in self-defense) and was soon caught, charged guilty with six death sentences, was put on death row for 10 years and then killed by lethal injection on October 9th, 2002 (Russell, 2002).

The nature of Wuornos' crimes highlight her complex psychological state. Her violent acts were not random but seemed to be driven by a deep-seated rage and a distorted perception of self-defense (Smith, 2011). The brutality and frequency of her attacks indicated a significant level of psychological distress and instability.

Psychological Profile

Aileen Wuornos, often referred to as "America's first female serial killer," offers a unique psychological profile that blends deeply rooted trauma, emotional turmoil, and a complex interplay of personality and environmental factors. Her story, often sensationalized in the media, raises important questions about the intersections of abuse, mental health, and criminality, challenging some of the traditional conceptions of serial killers, especially in terms of gender.

Aileen Carol Wuornos was born on February 29, 1956, in Rochester, Michigan, into a highly dysfunctional family. Her early years were marred by violence, neglect, and abandonment. Her father, who she never met, was a convicted sex offender who committed suicide in prison. When Aileen was just 4 years old, her mother abandoned her and her brother, leaving them in the care of their maternal grandparents. This household, however, was far from safe. Wuornos reportedly suffered physical, emotional, and sexual abuse at the hands of her grandfather, who was both violent and authoritarian. In addition to familial abuse, she experienced significant peer rejection and bullying during her childhood, further isolating her from sources of support and stability (Reynolds, 2016).

In psychological terms, Wuornos' childhood aligns closely with what is known as Adverse Childhood Experiences (ACEs), which are strongly correlated with an increased likelihood of various mental health issues, substance abuse, and criminal behavior later in life. Research has shown that early trauma, especially sustained trauma from trusted caregivers, often leads to insecure attachment styles, difficulties in regulating emotions, and an impaired ability to trust others. These developmental disruptions likely shaped her view of the world as a hostile, untrustworthy place, fostering a mindset where survival required constant self-defense and aggression.

Several psychological assessments and reports have suggested that Wuornos exhibited symptoms of borderline personality disorder (BPD), antisocial personality disorder (ASPD), and post-traumatic stress disorder (PTSD). Each of these disorders contributed uniquely to her psychological profile and to her criminal actions.

BPD is characterized by an intense fear of abandonment, emotional instability, impulsivity, and unstable relationships. Throughout her life, Wuornos displayed behaviors indicative of BPD, such as her volatile and short-lived romantic relationships, mood swings, and intense reactions to perceived rejection. She struggled with a chronic sense of emptiness and a fluctuating self-image, often swinging between idealization and devaluation of the people around her. Her relationships with men, in particular, were marked by distrust and hostility, likely fueled by her early abuse and exploitation.

ASPD involves a persistent pattern of disregard for the rights of others, often accompanied by manipulative, deceitful, and aggressive behaviors. Wuornos' criminal record, which began in her teenage years, included offenses such as robbery, assault, and fraud, all indicative of ASPD traits. Her lack of remorse and justification for her actions aligns with ASPD features. She often rationalized her killings by portraying herself as a victim acting in self-defense, even when the evidence contradicted her claims. Her repeated law-breaking, coupled with her disregard for societal norms, exemplifies ASPD, especially as it is expressed within the context of a highly troubled life.

Wuornos' history of severe abuse and trauma likely contributed to PTSD, with symptoms including hypervigilance, intrusive thoughts, and a strong startle response. These symptoms can heighten a person's perception of threat and make them more likely to react with aggression or violence, especially in situations perceived as threatening or hostile. Her claims that her victims had assaulted or attempted to harm her before she killed them may reflect an exaggerated perception of threat rooted in PTSD. This heightened sense of danger would have compounded her existing personality disorders, intensifying her aggressive responses.

Wuornos' experiences of abuse, rejection, and poverty fostered a hostile worldview where she saw life as a continuous struggle for survival. Her prolonged exposure to instability and betrayal likely contributed to a "survival mode" mentality, where she felt perpetually on guard against potential threats. This worldview was evident in her criminal lifestyle, which included substance abuse, sex work, and violence. Her self-reported view of men, in particular, was colored by resentment and anger, seeing them as exploitative and abusive figures. Such a perspective is consistent with research suggesting that trauma survivors often develop negative worldviews, leading to a tendency to misinterpret others' intentions, particularly in situations involving conflict.

For Wuornos, the unpredictable life of a sex worker also compounded her already high level of distrust and hostility. Her occupation placed her in vulnerable and dangerous situations, which could evoke a "fight or flight" response, especially for someone with PTSD and ASPD traits. Her decision to murder her clients, rather than flee, reflects both her impaired decision-making abilities and a distorted perception of these encounters as life-threatening situations.

Wuornos' murders followed a pattern wherein she targeted male clients who had solicited her services as a sex worker. In interviews and confessions, she repeatedly claimed that her actions were motivated by self-defense, insisting that her victims had either threatened or assaulted her. However, investigators and psychological experts questioned this narrative, citing inconsistencies and evidence that suggested many of the murders were premeditated rather than impulsive acts of self-defense.

Her justification aligns with a cognitive distortion often found in individuals with ASPD, where they externalize blame and rationalize their behavior to avoid taking responsibility. Wuornos' self-perception as a victim, even while committing violent crimes, may have provided a psychological buffer that allowed her to avoid the cognitive dissonance that would typically arise from such actions. She consistently framed her narrative to paint herself as a victim of an abusive and unfair world, enabling her to maintain a sense of moral righteousness even while engaging in horrific acts.

Impact of Mental Illness on Her Death Row Behavior

After her arrest and conviction, Wuornos' mental state deteriorated significantly. Her behavior on death row became erratic, and she exhibited increasingly paranoid delusions, believing that prison staff and others were conspiring against her. She also accused the media, her legal team, and even the judicial system of collusion. These behaviors suggest a possible progression of her mental illnesses, with her paranoia becoming more pronounced and her ability to differentiate reality from her fears diminishing.

This decline is characteristic of individuals with severe, untreated mental health conditions, particularly those exacerbated by isolation and stress. Her behavior on death row also raises ethical questions about the treatment of mentally ill prisoners, particularly in high-stress environments where symptoms can escalate without proper intervention.

Aileen Wuornos' psychological profile is complex, blending elements of borderline and antisocial personality traits, severe trauma, and environmental adversity. Her case reflects the deep scars left by abuse and abandonment and the powerful influence of untreated mental illness on behavior. Wuornos is an example of how mental health, personality disorders, and life circumstances can coalesce to drive individuals toward extreme actions, and her story highlights the need for better understanding and intervention in cases of severe childhood trauma and adult psychopathology. Her life and crimes remain a haunting reminder of the impact of unaddressed trauma and the often-tragic consequences of a life lived in survival mode.

Possible Treatment

Addressing Wuornos' psychological issues would have been extremely challenging. Cognitive-behavioral therapy (CBT) and trauma-focused therapies could have potentially helped manage her PTSD and BPD. However, the severity of her conditions and her resistance to authority would have posed significant obstacles to effective treatment (Arrigo & Griffin, 2004).

Given Wuornos' complex psychological profile, a comprehensive treatment approach involving a combination of therapeutic modalities and support services would have been necessary. However, the extent of her trauma and psychological disorders likely limited the potential effectiveness of these interventions (Foster, 2000).

Captivation and Trial

Wuornos was apprehended in January 1991 after a nationwide manhunt. Her arrest followed the discovery of her involvement in multiple murders, with evidence linking her to the crimes. During her trial, Wuornos initially claimed that she had acted in self-defense but later confessed to the murders. Her defense team argued that her severe psychological disorders should mitigate her culpability (Russell, 2002).

Wuornos was convicted and sentenced to death in 1992. She was executed by lethal injection in 2002. Her case drew significant media attention and sparked debates about mental illness, criminal responsibility, and the treatment of female offenders in the criminal justice system (Hickey, 2016; Smith, 2011).

Conclusion

The case of Aileen Wuornos underscores the tragic consequences of severe trauma and psychological disorders. Her background of abuse and neglect, combined with her psychological profile, provides crucial insights into the factors that drive individuals to commit violent crimes. Wuornos' life and criminal behavior highlight the urgent need for early intervention and effective treatment for those suffering from severe mental health issues.

Wuornos' story serves as a poignant reminder of the intersection between personal tragedy and criminal behavior. Understanding her psychological profile and the factors leading to her crimes can inform better approaches to preventing and addressing similar cases in the future (Arrigo & Griffin, 2004; McCord & McCord, 1964).

Aileen Wuornos poses as the prime example of a serial killer whose murderous tendencies can be solely attributed to the biological, psychological, and social factors of her years growing up. The abuse and trauma she went through at such a young age made her a vulnerable target to developing ASPD and attainting the label of a psychopath. Although she did begin with a biological predisposition to psychopathology, her tumultuous emotional states, violence, intense craving for power and deep-seated hatred for society collectively led to the creation of a serial killer.

References

Arrigo, B. A., & Griffin, A. (2004). Serial murder and the case of Aileen Wuornos: Attachment theory, psychopathy, and predatory aggression. *Behavioral Sciences & the Law*, *22*(3), 375–393.

Bartol, C. R., & Bartol, A. M. (2014). Current perspectives in forensic psychology and criminal Behavior. SAGE Publications.

Blonigen, D. M., Hicks, B. M., Krueger, R. F., Patrick, C. J., & Iacono, W. G. (2005). Psychopathic personality traits: Heritability and genetic overlap with internalizing and externalizing psychopathology. *Psychological Medicine*, *35*(5), 637–648.

Foster, D. (2000). *Monster: My true story*. Vision.

Hickey, E. W. (2016). *Serial murderers and their victims* (7th ed.). Cengage Learning.

Macleod, M. (2014). *Aileen Wuornos: Killer who preyed on truck drivers*. Retrieved from Crime library: https://www.crimelibrary.org/notorious_murders/women/wuornos/2.html.
McCord, W., & McCord, J. (1964). *The psychopath: An essay on the criminal mind*. Prentice-Hall.
Myers, W. C., Gooch, E., & Meloy, J. R. (2005). The role of psychopathy and sexuality in a female serial killer. *Journal of Forensic Sciences*, *50*(3), JFS2004324.
Pinel, J. P. (2014). Biopsychology (8th ed.). London: Pearson Allyn & Bacon.
Russell, S. (2002). *Damsel of death: Inside the mind of Aileen Wuornos*. Metro Publishing.
Smith, D. (2011). *Aileen Wuornos: The life and crimes of a female serial killer*. Palgrave Macmillan.
Reynolds, J. M. (2016). *Dead ends: The pursuit, conviction, and execution of serial killer Aileen Wuornos*. Open Road Media.

13

CASE STUDY OF JOACHIM KROLL

Introduction

Joachim Kroll, infamously known as the Ruhr Cannibal, stands as one of the most notorious serial killers in German history. Active from 1955 to 1976, Kroll's grisly acts of necrophilia and cannibalism shocked both the public and the psychological community (Martingale, 2015). This chapter delves into Kroll's psychological profile, the nature of his criminal behavior, and the underlying factors that fueled his heinous acts.

Background

Joachim Kroll was born on April 23, 1933, in Lipperland, Germany, at the end of World War I. His early life was characterized by poverty and familial instability. His father was abusive, while his mother was excessively overprotective, creating a tumultuous and dysfunctional home environment. These early experiences of violence and neglect significantly shaped Kroll's psychological development (Voss, 1990).

Kroll's childhood was marked by troubling behaviors, including setting fires and harming animals. He was also a bedwetter, which, with the above-mentioned two characteristics, form the McDonald triad. He struggled with severe learning disabilities and social isolation, which further alienated him from his peers and contributed to his growing sense of detachment. He had a borderline IQ of about 78 (tested later), and also reportedly low self-esteem as an adolescent (Bennett, 1997). By his teenage years, Kroll's psychological distress began manifesting in increasingly violent behaviors, setting the stage for his later criminal activities (Günther, 1984).

DOI: 10.4324/9781003602927-16

Kroll's upbringing took place in a low socio-economic environment, which can significantly impact personality and behavior. His family lived in poverty, and his childhood was marked by deprivation and neglect. Growing up in a large family with limited parental support, Kroll reportedly experienced physical and emotional isolation. Studies show that children from such backgrounds are more likely to develop maladaptive behaviors, especially when their familial environment lacks positive role models (Widom, 1989). Kroll's estrangement from social norms may have been partly due to his family's instability and the absence of a nurturing figure, which can hinder a child's understanding of societal boundaries (Hare, 1993).

Kroll was not good with his studies and repeated his classes multiple times, leading to him being in fourth grade at the age of 15. When he was a teen, World War II broke out, worsening his living conditions. He lost his father to World War II. He dropped out of school and started working as a butcher on his family farm. He reportedly was aroused by butchering. He also reported later that he was attached to his mother, and he stayed with her till her death. He became intrigued by death after his mother passed away. He separated from his siblings after his mother's death (Martingale, 2015).

Criminal Behavior

Kroll's killing spree commenced in the mid-1950s and continued until his arrest in 1976. Over this period, he was convicted of 14 murders, although he confessed to numerous additional killings. His modus operandi involved luring young women and children to isolated areas, where he would sexually assault, murder, and engage in acts of necrophilia and cannibalism (Krebs, 1978).

His first victim was a 19-year-old runaway, Irmgrad Stehl, whom he strangled to death. He committed necrophilia with her corpse and disemboweled her post-mortem. With his third victim, Frieda Tresman, who was murdered similarly to Stehl, he escalated to consuming the flesh of his victims. Most of his victims were girls and young women whose ages ranged from 4 to 24 years and were murdered and cannibalized. He had one male victim, 25-year-old Hermann Schmitz, who was attacked when he was having sex with a girl in his car. He was stabbed twice and was not sexually assaulted or cannibalized. He also had a 61-year-old victim who was stabbed and sexually assaulted but not cannibalized. His last and youngest victim was 4-year-old Marion Ketter whom he kidnapped from a park. Kroll had confessed that his cannibalism was related to supplementing his food with meat as he did not have money to buy meat otherwise (Martingale, 2015).

Kroll's crimes were marked by extreme brutality and a specific pattern of behavior. He targeted vulnerable victims, often from disadvantaged backgrounds, and used his cannibalistic tendencies as a means of exerting control and expressing profound psychological distress. Forensic investigations revealed that Kroll retained body parts from his victims, consuming them as part of his ritualistic behaviors (Bennett, 1997).

Psychological Profile

Joachim Kroll, often referred to as the "Ruhr Cannibal" or "The Duisburg Man-Eater," was a German serial killer and cannibal who murdered at least 14 people between 1955 and 1976 (Martingale, 2015). Kroll's crimes, rooted in deep psychological and emotional dysfunctions, reveal a complex profile of severe personality disorders, paraphilic disorders, and developmental impairments. Through exploring his behavioral patterns, cognitive functioning, emotional responses, and life history, we gain insights into how Kroll's disturbed psyche developed and manifested in such brutal acts.

Kroll was born in 1933 in Hindenburg, Germany (now Zabrze, Poland), as the youngest of eight children. His family endured extreme poverty, exacerbated by the effects of World War II and post-war conditions. Reports suggest that Kroll's father was abusive, further adding to the challenging environment in which he grew up (Bennett, 1997). Early experiences of neglect, deprivation, and possibly physical abuse can be considered contributing factors in the development of maladaptive coping mechanisms and attachment deficits.

In his early years, Kroll exhibited signs of developmental delays. His cognitive functioning appeared significantly below average, with an IQ reported to be around 76, which falls within the borderline intellectual functioning range (Bennett, 1997). His intellectual limitations affected his ability to connect socially, academically, and emotionally with his peers, likely exacerbating feelings of isolation and inferiority. The combination of a challenging home environment, cognitive limitations, and social rejection set the stage for the emergence of antisocial and disturbed tendencies. Psychologists and criminologists have proposed that Kroll exhibited signs consistent with several psychological disorders. A key element in his personality was an apparent deficiency in empathy and remorse, hallmark traits of antisocial personality disorder (ASPD). While some individuals with ASPD can be charming or manipulative, Kroll lacked social sophistication and instead exhibited overtly deviant behaviors that may be more associated with a schizoid or schizotypal presentation. His inability to form normal emotional connections and the lack of apparent distress over his crimes reveal a pervasive detachment from societal norms and expectations.

Additionally, Kroll's crimes involved acts of cannibalism, which suggest the presence of paraphilic disorders. He later admitted to consuming parts of his victims to save on grocery bills, a statement indicating not only a bizarre rationalization but also a severely disturbed view of human relationships (Bennett, 1997). This act of cannibalism likely reflects elements of necrophilic and anthropophagous fantasies, wherein Kroll achieved a sense of control or fulfillment by consuming his victims. His detachment from conventional morality allowed him to dehumanize his victims entirely, treating them as mere objects for satisfaction of his needs. Kroll's low cognitive functioning profoundly affected his judgment, impulse control, and capacity to anticipate consequences. His planning of the crimes was minimal; he often acted opportunistically and was driven by momentary impulses. His lack of sophistication in avoiding detection can be partially attributed to his limited cognitive capacity, which made him unable to fully comprehend or anticipate the repercussions of his actions. However, he demonstrated a rudimentary awareness of right and wrong, as seen in his attempts to hide evidence or flee the crime scenes. This partial understanding indicates that while he may have had limited cognitive resources, he was not wholly ignorant of societal laws and consequences.

In interviews, Kroll described how he learned from each crime to avoid mistakes, suggesting that he was capable of a rudimentary form of procedural learning. His approach to killing was repetitive and patterned, indicating that he felt compelled to return to similar methods and tactics. However, the cognitive rigidity he demonstrated, combined with his limited ability to adapt in a more complex manner, ultimately contributed to his capture.

An important dimension of Kroll's profile involves the fantasies that fueled his motivations. His confessions revealed a fascination with power, control, and gratification achieved through violence, suggesting a disturbed sexual-sadistic orientation. His crimes often involved sexual assault, which may have served as a means to exert dominance, thereby compensating for his lack of control in other areas of life. This compulsive need for control over others aligns with traits seen in paraphilic and personality disorders, where gratification is achieved through harming others, leading to a cycle of dependency on such behaviors for emotional release. Cannibalism added another layer to Kroll's pathology. His motivations were not purely economic, despite his claims about saving on food expenses. The consumption of his victims can be interpreted as a symbolic act of ultimate possession and destruction, wherein he assimilated his victims, achieving a perverse form of intimacy through ingestion. This aligns with the extreme dehumanization of his victims, whom he saw as extensions of his needs and desires rather than as independent individuals.

Kroll's limited social network and his interpersonal ineptitude reveal another dimension of his psychological dysfunction. Described as a loner by neighbors and co-workers, he maintained a low social profile, with minimal engagement in community life. His stunted social skills further isolated him, depriving him of any meaningful emotional bonds or corrective feedback from others. Isolation is often a critical risk factor in criminality, particularly in individuals with disturbed personalities, as it fosters rumination and fixation on deviant thoughts. Interestingly, Kroll appeared to maintain a superficial appearance of normalcy, working at a factory and interacting minimally with neighbors, suggesting he possessed some basic social adaptation skills.

This low-level adaptation might have allowed him to avoid suspicion for an extended period, yet his fundamentally dysfunctional approach to relationships kept him disconnected from any social norms that might have mitigated his behavior.

Kroll's arrest in 1976 followed the disappearance of a 4-year-old girl, whom he had abducted, killed, and partially consumed (Bennett, 1997). During interrogation, Kroll readily confessed to his crimes without signs of guilt or distress, even providing details of his cannibalistic acts with apparent indifference. His lack of remorse and emotional detachment during confession reflect severe emotional blunting and suggest the presence of schizoid characteristics. Psychological evaluations conducted post-arrest pointed to an impoverished inner world, a tendency toward isolation, and deeply ingrained deviant sexual preferences. Kroll's straightforward and detached confessions illustrated his dissociation from normal human empathy and an inability to understand his own motivations, a symptom commonly seen in individuals with severe personality and psychotic disorders.

Joachim Kroll's psychological profile is a confluence of cognitive limitations, personality pathology, paraphilic tendencies, and severe detachment from societal norms. His intellectual impairments hindered his ability to process moral standards, while his profound lack of empathy allowed him to treat others as objects. His development of deviant fantasies, compounded by social isolation and an inability to form healthy relationships, fostered a life driven by compulsive, violent behavior. Kroll's case illustrates how severe developmental, cognitive, and personality dysfunctions can intertwine to form a pathological identity and a lethal disregard for human life.

Possible Treatment

Treating individuals with Kroll's psychological profile presents substantial challenges. Given his severe antisocial tendencies and psychopathic traits, traditional therapeutic approaches such as cognitive-behavioral therapy (CBT) may have limited effectiveness. Kroll's lack of remorse and emotional detachment would likely hinder the success of conventional treatment methods (Günther, 1984).

In cases involving severe psychopathy and entrenched criminal behavior, a multidisciplinary approach combining psychiatric treatment with strict behavioral monitoring might be necessary. However, the extent of Kroll's psychological disorders and his entrenched patterns of violence would have made effective treatment exceptionally difficult (Bennett, 1997).

Captivation and Trial

Joachim Kroll was apprehended in 1976 after a prolonged investigation that connected him to several unsolved murders. The breakthrough in his capture came from forensic evidence found in his residence, linking him conclusively to the crimes. Post the missing of his last victim Marion Ketter, the police started searching the neighborhood. After receiving complaints of a clogged drain by a tenant in Kroll's apartment, police checked the drainage of the apartment where they found human intestines. Later, on raiding Kroll's apartment, police found rest of the body parts in his refrigerator. His drainage pipes were clogged with body parts and a hand was found cooking on his stove. During his trial, Kroll displayed a chilling lack of remorse and a detached demeanor, further unsettling the public and the judicial system (Krebs, 1978).

Kroll was convicted of multiple counts of murder and sentenced to life imprisonment. He died in 1991 while serving his sentence. His case underscored the challenges of understanding and treating individuals with severe psychological disorders and highlighted the importance of forensic psychology in criminal investigations (Günther, 1984).

Conclusion

The case of Joachim Kroll illustrates the intricate relationship between severe psychological disorders and violent criminal behavior. His background of abuse, combined with his psychopathic traits, provides crucial insights into the motivations behind his horrific actions. Kroll's story serves as a stark reminder of the need for comprehensive psychological assessment and intervention in cases of extreme criminal behavior.

Understanding Kroll's psychological profile and the factors contributing to his crimes can inform better strategies for preventing and addressing similar cases in the future. His case emphasizes the importance of forensic psychology in comprehending and managing individuals with severe psychological disturbances (Voss, 1990; Bennett, 1997).

References

Bennett, T. (1997). *The psychology of serial killers: Exploring the mind of the Ruhr Cannibal*. HarperCollins.

Günther, M. (1984). *The anatomy of evil: Psychopathology and criminal behavior*. Springer.

Hare, R. D. (1993). Without conscience: The disturbing world of the psychopaths among us. Beyond Words/Atria Books.

Krebs, C. (1978). *Inside the mind of a cannibal: The case of Joachim Kroll*. Routledge.

Martingale, M. (2015). *Cannibal killers: The Impossible Monsters*. Quetzalcoatl Publishing. 10.75.

Voss, H. (1990). *Joachim Kroll: The Ruhr Cannibal and the psychology of deviance*. Cambridge University Press.

Widom, C. S. (1989). The cycle of violence. *Science, 244*(4901), 160–166. https://doi.org/10.1126/science.2704995

PART IV

Familial Crimes and Psychological Motivations

14

CASE STUDY ON THE MENENDEZ BROTHERS

Introduction

The case of Lyle and Erik Menendez is a compelling study in forensic psychology involving the brutal murder of their parents and a highly publicized trial that brought their history of abuse into the spotlight. This chapter delves into the Menendez brothers' background, their criminal behavior, their psychological profile, and the implications of their case for understanding the relationship between trauma and criminal conduct.

Background

Lyle and Erik Menendez were born in the early 1970s to Jose and Kitty Menendez, a wealthy couple living in Beverly Hills, California. Despite the family's affluence, the brothers' upbringing was marred by severe emotional and physical abuse. According to trial testimonies and psychological evaluations, the Menendez brothers faced ongoing sexual abuse by their father, Jose Menendez, along with physical violence from both parents (Benedict, 1995; Berkowitz, 1996).

Jose and Kitty Menendez met in college, got married, and moved to New York. Jose Menendez worked as an accountant and Kitty Menendez was a teacher. They gave birth to their first son, Joseph Lyle Menendez aka Lyle, in 1968 and their second son Erik Galen Mendez in 1970. Jose Menendez secured a high-paying job in an accounting firm. Kitty Menendez quit her job as a teacher and the Menendez family moved to Illinois. Jose Menendez was fired from this job and was hired by another firm after a short while. Lyle

DOI: 10.4324/9781003602927-18

Menendez reported later that his mother was happy during the early years of the marriage, but the money did not do good for their parents' marriage (Rand, 2018).

Relatives describe the Menendez brothers to be mischievous during their childhood. Jose Menendez was often controlling about the brothers not having playmates of their age as he claimed that it would distract the boys. He was reported to have been physically violent with the children. Kitty Menendez too did not show much affection toward the brothers and was reported to have verbally abused and thrown things at them. Lyle Menendez was encouraged to bully his brother by Jose Menendez. Jose Menendez also encouraged the two brothers to be disrespectful to their mother. The Menendezes were strict parents who expected that their children excel in both academic and sports activities (Rand, 2018).

The family moved to California after Jose Menendez secured a position as an executive at Hertz corporation. Jose Menendez had at least two extramarital affairs, which were discovered by his wife. Their relationship became more chaotic, which affected the children. Jose Menendez became more and more demanding on Lyle and Eric. Jose and Kitty Menendez even tried to hide the suspension of Lyle Menendez from Princeton University because of a plagiarism of assignment. Lyle and Eric Menendez were caught in a burglary, which they committed with a group of friends in 1988 (Rand, 2018).

The Menendez family had more secrets that emerged when Lyle and Eric Menendez were facing trial for their parents' murders. Lyle Menendez reported that his father had sexually abused him when he was 6 years old to 8 years old. Eric Menendez reported that his father's next victim was himself, and he was sexually abused by his father from the age of 6 to adulthood. The brothers also reported that their mother was a neglectful parent who had problems with alcohol and drugs. They also reported that their mother was aware of the abuse but never stopped their father (Mulvey, Fournier, & Donahue, 2006).

Their privileged exterior concealed a deeply troubled home environment characterized by manipulation, control, and secrecy. The brothers' experiences of abuse were compounded by the pressure to maintain the façade of a perfect family. This toxic environment created a context in which the brothers' psychological development was profoundly affected, contributing to their eventual criminal actions (Benedict, 1995; Millon, Simonsen, Birket-Smith, & Davis, 2010).

Criminal Behavior

On August 20, 1989, Lyle and Erik Menendez carried out the brutal murder of their parents, Jose and Kitty Menendez, in their Beverly Hills home. The brothers executed their plan with premeditation, using shotguns to kill their parents in a violent attack that was initially staged to look like a burglary gone wrong. The prosecution argued that the murders were motivated by the brothers' desire for their parents' wealth and financial security. In contrast, the defense presented a case of abuse, claiming that the murders were an act of desperation rooted in long-standing trauma and fear (Benedict, 1995; Bodine, 1994).

In the trials Eric Menendez reported that he had told his brother about the sexual abuse inflicted on them by their father. The brothers then proceeded to confront their parents with this information, and were allegedly threatened by their father. They then proceeded to buy shotguns claiming that the guns were for self-protection. On the night of the murders, Jose and Kitty Menendez were watching a movie in their living room. Witnesses reported that they had seen two men in a vehicle heading toward the Menendez home. The brothers first killed Jose Menendez, firing multiple shots at him. Kitty Menendez was also shot at but she managed to crawl toward the door. The brothers went out and reloaded the gun with bird shots and fired at their mother, killing her. They then proceeded to go out and wait for someone to discover the crime scene. However, when they returned the following day expecting police at their doorsteps, they were disappointed to see that no one has reported the crime. They then proceeded to call the police themselves and reported the murders (Mulvey et al., 2006).

The case became a media sensation, and the trial provided a dramatic portrayal of the brothers' troubled past. The detailed accounts of the abuse and the brothers' psychological states were crucial in shaping public perception and the legal outcome of the trial (Berkowitz, 1996).

Psychological Profile

The Menendez brothers, Lyle and Erik, became infamous for the brutal 1989 murder of their parents, José and Kitty Menendez, in their Beverly Hills mansion (Mulvey et al., 2006). The case drew significant media attention and sparked widespread public fascination and controversy. Understanding the psychological profiles of Lyle and Erik Menendez requires delving into their upbringing, the nature of their family dynamics, the reported abuse they endured, and the mental and emotional toll of their family environment. Their case highlights complex themes of power, control, trauma, and the impact of long-term abuse on behavior and decision-making.

Lyle and Erik were raised in a wealthy, high-achieving family, but one that reportedly maintained strict, authoritarian dynamics. José Menendez, a successful entertainment executive, was known to be domineering and exacting, imposing severe expectations on his sons. Kitty Menendez was described as emotionally fragile, dependent, and largely passive in the family's decision-making structure, often yielding to José's authority. While the family enjoyed financial privilege, the environment within the home was reportedly one of rigidity, high pressure, and emotional isolation (Mulvey et al., 2006).

Friends and acquaintances later recalled the Menendez home as outwardly luxurious but lacking warmth. Lyle and Erik were conditioned to uphold the family's public image and were reportedly pressured to excel, particularly in sports and academics, to align with José's standards of perfection. This external pressure, combined with their lack of close friends or confidantes, left the brothers increasingly isolated and reliant on each other for emotional support. A central component of the Menendez brothers' psychological profiles involves the allegations of prolonged abuse. During their trial, both Lyle and Erik claimed that they had endured years of sexual, physical, and psychological abuse at the hands of their father. Lyle testified that José subjected them to violent and dehumanizing treatment, which included beatings and threats, while Kitty reportedly turned a blind eye, out of either fear or dependence on José.

The abuse claims form the foundation of their defense and significantly influence their psychological profiles. Prolonged abuse can lead to complex trauma, often resulting in significant issues such as dissociation, attachment difficulties, feelings of helplessness, low self-esteem, and heightened sensitivity to stressors. The brothers' descriptions of their abuse are consistent with symptoms often seen in victims of complex trauma, including hypervigilance, feelings of entrapment, and a diminished sense of autonomy. Erik, who was younger and reportedly more submissive, appeared to internalize the trauma more deeply than Lyle, possibly contributing to greater emotional volatility and vulnerability to influence from his older brother.

While Lyle and Erik shared common trauma, their personalities and roles within the family hierarchy reveal distinct psychological traits. Lyle, the elder brother, appeared to adopt a more protective, controlling role. Witnesses and family members described Lyle as the more dominant and assertive of the two, traits which likely developed as coping mechanisms in an attempt to shield both himself and Erik from their father's authoritarianism. Lyle's personality is marked by traits often associated with those forced into a caregiving or defensive role early in life, including increased impulsivity, a need to exert control, and occasional aggression.

In contrast, Erik displayed characteristics of a more submissive, emotionally sensitive personality. He reportedly idolized his older brother and depended on Lyle for support and decision-making, suggesting a bond shaped by dependency rather than equality. Erik's emotional fragility and susceptibility to Lyle's influence made him more vulnerable to emotional manipulation. He exhibited signs of anxiety and emotional instability, which may be explained by his difficulty coping with the trauma independently. During the trial, Erik appeared more openly remorseful, tearful, and guilt-ridden than Lyle, further underscoring his heightened emotional sensitivity. The Menendez brothers' decision to kill their parents can be viewed through the lens of long-term trauma and the psychological impact of severe power imbalances. Their account suggested that they saw no viable escape from their abusive situation and experienced overwhelming feelings of entrapment. For individuals subjected to prolonged abuse, psychological mechanisms such as "learned helplessness" and hypervigilance can foster a distorted perception of their reality, wherein drastic solutions seem necessary for survival.

Psychologists have posited that the decision to murder their parents may have stemmed from a shared psychotic disorder, or "folie à deux," in which Erik's dependency on Lyle reinforced a shared worldview and psychological justification for their actions. Their intense reliance on each other, coupled with shared trauma, could have created an echo chamber of distorted thinking, wherein their fear, desperation, and anger escalated into homicidal intent. In such cases, the more dominant personality, Lyle, might drive decision-making while the more submissive party, Erik, becomes complicit, seeking validation from the more assertive sibling.

While the brothers contended that abuse was their primary motive, their critics argue that financial gain was also a significant factor. After the murder, Lyle and Erik engaged in extravagant spending, which raised questions about whether greed and entitlement played a role in their decision. From a psychological standpoint, the financial behavior exhibited after the murders may reflect a combination of disinhibition and delayed gratification resulting from years of repression and trauma. Their spending could also indicate a subconscious need to reclaim control and assert their newfound autonomy, a stark departure from years of financial dependency and domination by their father.

The question of whether financial gain was a primary or secondary motivator is further complicated by the abuse allegations. Financial motivations do not negate the presence of trauma and abuse; rather, they might represent a complex interplay between the desire for freedom, control, and a tangible reward for years of suffering. In abusive situations, victims sometimes come to view wealth or material possessions as symbols of liberation, as they represent both physical and psychological independence from their abusers. Following their arrest, the psychological profiles of Lyle and Erik were further revealed in their responses to interrogation, trial proceedings, and incarceration. Erik displayed pronounced remorse and emotional breakdowns during the trial, indicating a strong awareness of guilt and possibly internalized shame. Lyle, while also expressing regret, appeared more controlled and assertive, occasionally adopting a defensive posture. These reactions align with their roles within the family and suggest differing levels of emotional processing and acceptance of guilt.

During the trial, their defense leaned heavily on the abuse allegations, aiming to contextualize their actions within the trauma they endured. Experts who evaluated the brothers described symptoms consistent with post-traumatic stress disorder (PTSD), complex trauma, and maladaptive coping mechanisms. These evaluations painted a picture of two individuals trapped in a cycle of fear and subjugation, culminating in an act they saw as both liberatory and retributive.

An intricate web of familial dysfunction, trauma, and individual personality dynamics shapes the Menendez brothers' psychological profiles. Lyle and Erik were subject to extreme parental control, emotional neglect, and possibly sustained abuse, leading to profound emotional and psychological scars. These experiences, combined with their contrasting personality traits, fostered a toxic dependency that led to mutual reinforcement of distorted thinking and, ultimately, violent action. Their case exemplifies the devastating impact of abuse and psychological isolation, demonstrating how unaddressed trauma can lead to extreme responses. While their financial actions post-murder remain controversial, their psychological profiles suggest that their actions were deeply rooted in a desperate need for control, freedom, and self-preservation. The Menendez case stands as a reminder of the profound effects of trauma on human behavior and the complex factors that drive individuals to commit heinous acts against those closest to them.

Possible Treatment

Addressing the psychological issues faced by Lyle and Erik Menendez would require a multifaceted approach. Trauma-focused cognitive-behavioral therapy (CBT) could be instrumental in treating their PTSD, aiming to process and reframe their traumatic experiences. Additionally, therapeutic interventions would focus on managing symptoms of depression and borderline personality traits, helping the individuals develop healthier coping strategies (Bodine, 1994; Millon et al., 2010).

However, the severity of their conditions and the complexity of their trauma would present significant challenges to treatment. Long-term psychological support and monitoring would be essential for addressing their deep-seated issues and facilitating their emotional healing (Holmes & Rahe, 1967).

Captivation and Trial

The police in the initial investigation determined that the murders were committed by someone who knew the Menendezes as there was no sign of breaking and entering. The Menedez brothers were able to give a detailed description of their whereabouts and were not initially considered suspects. But their extravagant spending weeks after their parents' death made them look suspicious. Backing this suspicion was Eric Menendez's confession to his friend and therapist. Eric Menendez had even written a screenplay weeks prior to the murders on how he would kill his parents. There were also reports of Lyle Mendez hiring a computer expert to erase the latest will of Jose Menendez, which would have given less assets to the brothers. The police arrested Lyle Menendez shortly and Eric Menendez surrendered himself three days later (Staff, 2024).

The Menendez brothers' trial was one of the most sensational and scrutinized legal cases of the 1990s. The defense's argument of abuse played a central role in the trial, with testimony from psychologists and family members providing insight into the brothers' traumatic past. The jury ultimately convicted Lyle and Erik Menendez of first-degree murder, and they were sentenced to life imprisonment without the possibility of parole (Benedict, 1995; Berkowitz, 1996).

The case remains a notable example of how psychological trauma can influence criminal behavior and the legal system's response to such cases. It underscores the importance of understanding the impact of abuse on individuals and the complexities of integrating psychological evidence into legal proceedings (Bodine, 1994).

Conclusion

The case of the Menendez brothers highlights the profound effects of psychological trauma and abuse on criminal behavior. Their tragic actions and the subsequent trial illustrate the interplay between severe emotional distress and criminal conduct. Understanding the Menendez brothers' psychological profile provides valuable insights into the factors driving such extreme behavior and underscores the necessity for effective mental health interventions and support for those experiencing significant trauma.

Their case serves as a critical reminder of the need for comprehensive psychological assessments in legal contexts and the importance of addressing trauma in preventing and managing severe criminal behavior (Millon et al., 2010; Berkowitz, 1996).

References

Benedict, A. (1995). *The Menendez brothers: The trial of the century*. St. Martin's Press.

Berkowitz, L. (1996). *Understanding aggression: The Menendez brothers case*. Academic Press.

Bodine, T. (1994). *The Menendez case: A study in trauma and criminal behavior*. Psychological Press.

Holmes, T. H., & Rahe, R. H. (1967). The social readjustment rating scale. *Journal of Psychosomatic Research*, *11*(2), 213–218.

Millon, T., Simonsen, E., Birket-Smith, M., & Davis, R. D. (2010). *Psychopathy: Antisocial, criminal, and violent behavior* (2nd ed.). Guilford Press.

Mulvey, A., Fournier, A., & Donahue, T. (2006). Murder in the family: The Menendez Brothers. *Victims & Offenders*, *1*(3), 213–224. https://doi.org/10.1080/15564880600843677

Rand, R. (2018). *The Menendez murders: The shocking untold story of the Menendez family and the killings that stunned the nation*. BenBella Books.

Staff, C. T. (2024, September 19). 59-CA v. Menendez: Erik Menendez (part 2). Court TV. https://www.courttv.com/title/59-ca-v-menendez-erik-menendez-pt2/

15

NITHARI SERIAL MURDER CASE

Introduction

The Nithari case, one of the most chilling and gruesome criminal investigations in recent Indian history, came to light in 2006. This chapter provides an in-depth analysis of the case, exploring the details of the horrific crimes committed, the psychological profiles of the perpetrators, and the forensic investigation that brought them to justice.

Background

In 2006, Nithari village near Noida was thrust into the spotlight when authorities uncovered a series of dismembered bodies buried in the backyard of a house belonging to Moninder Singh Pandher and Surinder Koli. The discovery of these bodies led to a nationwide outcry and revealed the extent of the heinous activities carried out by the perpetrators. Surinder Koli, an employee of Pandher, and Pandher himself were implicated in the kidnapping, sexual assault, and murder of children and young women. The investigation unveiled a chilling pattern of violence and exploitation that had been ongoing for several years (Sharma, 2009).

Koli and Pandher's victims were primarily from impoverished backgrounds, making them vulnerable to exploitation. The perpetrators used various means to lure their victims to Pandher's house, where they were subjected to brutal treatment. The severity of the crimes committed shocked both the public and the authorities, highlighting severe lapses in law enforcement and child protection mechanisms (Singh, 2008).

DOI: 10.4324/9781003602927-19

The primary accused in the case was Surinder Koli, the domestic help of the affluent businessman and Koli's alleged partner in crime Moninder Singh Pandher. Koli hails from a remote village in Almora district of Uttarakhand. He dropped out of school after completing his sixth standard. There are reports of Koli being sexually abused and bullied by older students when he was a child. After dropping out of school, Koli did odd jobs and worked in a hotel. He moved to Delhi in search of better opportunities and worked as a cook at the home of a retired brigadier in Noida for 5 years. He left his job in 1998 and went back to his village to get married. He had two children with his wife, a son and a daughter. He left his wife and went back to Noida, where he worked for an army major for 6 months. He was then recommended to Panther and worked in Pandher's now infamous D5 Bungalow in Sector 31 Noida, till he was caught in 2006 (Blanco, n.d.).

The co-accused in the Nithari case, Moninder Singh Pandher, was a well-known businessman, who inherited his wealth from his father. He was well educated and described as a steady chap by his friends and colleagues. He was married with a son, but was estranged from both his wife and his son and lived alone in his Noida home. He was addicted to alcohol and had a luxurious lifestyle. There were also reports of Pandher allegedly encountering sexual assault as a child (Blanco, n.d.).

Criminal Behavior

The Nithari case was marked by extreme brutality and systematic violence. Koli and Pandher's criminal activities included the abduction of their victims, who were then sexually assaulted, murdered, and dismembered. The perpetrators exhibited a disturbing level of premeditation and organization in their crimes. They would lure victims with promises of employment or other benefits, only to trap them in a nightmarish scenario.

The dismemberment of bodies was a particularly gruesome aspect of their crimes, reflecting a complete disregard for human life and an attempt to conceal evidence. The forensic investigation revealed that the murders were not random but part of a horrifying pattern of behavior, with Koli and Pandher meticulously planning and executing their criminal activities (Sharma, 2009).

Koli started abducting children from Nithari village in 2004, when he coerced a small girl, Rimpa Haldar, strangled her, and cooked and consumed her breast. He similarly killed and cannibalized at least 19 young victims. The police estimated that the number of victims might be over 30, but no remains were found to link Koli to these cases. Koli also had an adult victim, a 20-year-old girl, Payal, with whom he had a sexual relationship under an alias. With Pandher, it is not known whether he had any connections with the crimes. Police, however, found it highly unlikely that Pandher was unaware of someone "killing, cutting and eating" children in his house. The popular theory was that Pandher and Koli were a team. Koli kidnapped the children and took them to Pandher who would sexually assault them. Koli would then proceed to kill and cannibalize them and dispose of their body (Blanco, n.d.).

Psychological Profile

Surinder Koli's background plays a critical role in understanding his actions and psychological state. Koli was born into a poor family in Uttarakhand, India. His early life was marked by poverty, deprivation, and a lack of stable family support. Little is known about any childhood abuse or trauma he may have endured, but the circumstances of extreme poverty, limited education, and a lack of parental nurturing likely had a significant impact on his psychological development.

Poverty and deprivation in childhood are known to increase risks for a range of psychological issues, including anxiety, depression, and impaired social functioning. For Koli, the challenges he faced growing up in a low-income, resource-deprived environment may have contributed to a sense of social isolation and mistrust of others, leading him to seek low-paying domestic work as a means of survival. Koli's migration to the city and subsequent employment with Pandher in Noida marked his first exposure to urban life, bringing with it new challenges, stresses, and frustrations.

Accounts of Koli's personality reveal him as a socially withdrawn and passive individual. Known to be quiet and submissive, Koli likely displayed avoidant or socially anxious traits, preferring to keep to himself and not engage much with others. Some reports suggest he had difficulty forming meaningful relationships, likely as a result of his early environment and socio-economic background, which could have fostered feelings of inadequacy and low self-worth.

Koli's apparent lack of social skills and tendency toward introversion may have led him to retreat further into isolation. Social isolation, coupled with his low social standing, could have created a psychological environment where he had few outlets for self-expression or emotional release. This isolation could have fostered deeply ingrained resentments and frustrations, which he may have lacked the tools to express in healthy ways. In some cases, extreme isolation and social deprivation can lead individuals to develop disturbing thoughts, fantasies, and even violent tendencies as a means of gaining control over their inner turmoil.

Given the severity and nature of Koli's crimes, some experts have speculated that he may have displayed traits consistent with psychopathy or other severe mental disorders. A lack of empathy, shallow emotions, impulsive behaviors, and an inclination toward antisocial activities characterizes psychopathy. While it's challenging to diagnose Koli without a direct psychological evaluation, his actions suggest a profound absence of remorse, empathy, or understanding of the moral gravity of his actions.

Psychopathy, or even antisocial personality disorder, would explain Koli's capacity to commit horrendous acts without apparent remorse. This absence of empathy and disregard for others' lives could point to a severe personality disorder. Reports indicate that Koli expressed disturbing fantasies, including cannibalistic urges and necrophilia, which align with behaviors associated with certain paraphilic disorders. His behavior reflects a clear detachment from societal norms and a lack of respect for human life, suggesting an inner world dominated by dark, uncontrollable impulses.

During the investigation, Koli confessed to experiencing disturbing and violent urges, including acts of necrophilia and cannibalism. These behaviors may be indicative of a paraphilic disorder, where an individual derives sexual or psychological gratification from atypical, often extreme, acts that are socially or morally unacceptable. Koli's actions point to a sadistic form of paraphilia, in which he derived pleasure or satisfaction from committing acts that involved power, control, and the complete dehumanization of his victims.

The combination of isolation, traumatic background, and the lack of healthy outlets for expression may have led Koli to develop these sadistic fantasies as a way to exercise control over his life. Some psychological theories suggest that individuals with certain types of paraphilia often feel powerless or invisible in their everyday lives, turning to extreme fantasies as a way to feel powerful or significant. For Koli, these dark fantasies may have provided a temporary release, though in a disturbingly violent and harmful manner.

Koli's modus operandi reflected a level of planning and control, which is typical of individuals with psychopathic tendencies. He would lure young children, usually those from poorer families who wouldn't be immediately missed, into the house under the guise of offering them something. Once inside, he would murder them, mutilate their bodies, and, in some cases, even consume parts of their remains.

Koli's actions suggest compulsive tendencies, meaning he may have felt an overwhelming need to carry out these horrific acts. Psychological compulsion often stems from an inability to resist urges or thoughts, and, for Koli, this compulsion may have become stronger over time, fueling his behavior in a self-reinforcing cycle. His actions grew more frequent, pointing to an escalating need to satisfy his dark impulses—a characteristic often observed in serial offenders.

The relationship between Koli and his employer, Moninder Singh Pandher, also warrants psychological consideration. Pandher's apparent control over Koli as an employer and the imbalanced power dynamic between them may have reinforced Koli's feelings of subjugation and powerlessness. Some have suggested that Koli may have initially harbored resentment toward Pandher, and his violent actions against the most vulnerable in society could have been a way to exert control where he otherwise felt powerless. This assertion remains speculative, yet it aligns with the psychological mechanism of displaced aggression, where pent-up anger or resentment is redirected toward others, often weaker or more vulnerable targets. Koli's lack of remorse or moral insight into his crimes points to a complete moral detachment. During interrogations, he showed a disturbing calmness and lack of regret, a characteristic trait of individuals with psychopathic tendencies. This moral detachment allowed him to dehumanize his victims and view them merely as objects to fulfill his compulsions.

The absence of guilt or emotional conflict highlights Koli's impaired empathy, which may stem from a combination of his traumatic upbringing, social isolation, and personality structure. Individuals with extreme antisocial tendencies often lack the internal moral framework that most people rely on to regulate behavior, and Koli's actions reflect an individual completely detached from the consequences of his actions.

Severe social isolation, possible psychopathic tendencies, and disturbing paraphilic disorders mark Surinder Koli's psychological profile. His tragic background of poverty and deprivation likely contributed to his inability to form meaningful social bonds, ultimately leading him to retreat into a world of sadistic fantasies and compulsive violence. Lacking empathy and moral grounding, Koli became capable of carrying out unimaginable acts, ultimately turning his psychological distress into violent, predatory behavior. The Nithari case underscores the critical importance of understanding the psychological backgrounds of offenders and the social conditions that may contribute to such extreme criminality. Koli's case remains a chilling example of how unaddressed trauma, deprivation, and psychological disorders can result in devastating consequences, revealing the complex interplay between personal history, psychological dysfunction, and horrific violence.

Possible Treatment

Effective treatment for individuals like Surinder Koli and Moninder Singh Pandher would require a comprehensive approach, combining psychiatric medication and intensive psychotherapy. For Koli, antipsychotic medications and therapy focusing on impulse control, empathy development, and addressing sadistic tendencies would be critical. For Pandher, therapy would need to address moral and psychological dysfunctions, aiming to foster a sense of responsibility and empathy. Continuous monitoring and rehabilitation programs could potentially mitigate the risk of reoffending, although the severity of their disorders poses significant challenges.

Captivation and Trial

The missing children of Nithari village were initially treated as runaways by police and no actions were taken by the police to find them. It wasn't until 2006 when villagers of Nithari found human remains in the municipal water tank behind Panther's house the police started investigating the missing as possible serial murders. Later that year, police brought in Panther and Koli for the missing case of Payal. Koli then started confessing about the gruesome murders he committed. The case was later handed over to the CBI for investigation (Blanco, n.d.).

The forensic investigation into the Nithari case was complex and involved multiple techniques to link Koli and Pandher to the crimes. Key aspects included:

Crime Scene Analysis: The examination of the crime scenes involved the recovery of dismembered body parts and the collection of DNA evidence, which was crucial in linking the perpetrators to the crimes (Singh, 2008).

DNA Analysis: Forensic DNA analysis played a pivotal role in confirming the identities of the victims and establishing a connection between the crimes and the suspects (Sharma, 2009).

Interrogation and Evidence: Detailed interrogation of Koli and Pandher, combined with the forensic evidence gathered, led to their confessions and subsequent convictions. The investigation highlighted the importance of forensic science in solving complex and heinous crimes (Sinha, 2020). The Nithari case resulted in the conviction of Surinder Koli and Moninder Singh Pandher, who were sentenced to life imprisonment. In a recent overturn of events, Pandher and Koli were both acquitted of charges where the Allahabad high court claimed that police had done a sloppy investigation with no real evidence connecting both accused to the crime. The case underscored significant issues in the criminal justice system, including the need for more effective child protection measures and improved law enforcement practices. It also highlighted the crucial role of forensic science in addressing and solving severe criminal cases (Singh, 2008; Sharma, 2009).

Conclusion

The Nithari case remains a stark reminder of the depths of human depravity and the challenges of addressing extreme violence. It underscores the need for comprehensive psychological assessments, effective forensic investigations, and robust legal frameworks to prevent and address similar cases. Understanding the psychological profiles and criminal behaviors of individuals involved in such horrific acts can provide valuable insights into preventing future tragedies and improving the criminal justice system.

References

Blanco, J. I. (n.d.). Surender Koli|Murderpedia, the encyclopedia of murderers. https://murderpedia.org/male.K/k/koli-surender.htm

Sharma, P. (2009). *The Nithari horror: A forensic analysis of the Noida killings*. Oxford University Press.

Singh, R. (2008). *The Nithari case: Forensic investigation and criminal justice*. Sage Publications.

Sinha, D. (2020). Narco-analysis test: Truth serum or torture. *International Journal of Law Management & Humanities*, *3*(2), 411.

16

THE CASEY ANTHONY TRIAL

Introduction

The Casey Anthony trial captured global attention with its dramatic courtroom battles and controversial verdicts. This chapter delves into the complexities of the case, examining Casey Anthony's psychological profile, her criminal behavior, and the factors that contributed to the highly debated acquittal.

Background

Casey Marie Anthony was born in Warren, Ohio, on March 19, 1986. Raised in a middle-class family, Anthony's early life seemed typical, but a series of troubling events began to unfold when her 2-year-old daughter, Caylee Anthony, went missing in July 2008. Caylee's disappearance led to a massive search effort, but her skeletal remains were found in December 2008 in a wooded area near the Anthony family home. The investigation into Caylee's death, coupled with Casey's erratic behavior, created a media frenzy and raised suspicions about her involvement in her daughter's death (Baden & Homicz, 2012; Perry, 2009).

The initial investigation revealed inconsistencies in Casey's accounts of Caylee's whereabouts. Her prolonged delay in reporting Caylee missing, coupled with her attempts to mislead investigators, fueled public and legal scrutiny. The case became a focal point for discussions on parental responsibility and legal standards in criminal investigations (Perry, 2009).

Anthony was described as a bright and friendly young girl. Her friends report that Anthony developed a habit of lying when she was in high school.

DOI: 10.4324/9781003602927-20

She had convinced her family that she had completed her high school education, when she was actually failing in her classes and even stopped attending school toward the semester end. Her parents and grandparents found that she had been lying to them when they went to her high school graduation. Later when she was 19, she was pregnant with Caylee, she initially refused to admit that she had been gaining weight because of pregnancy. She named many men as Caylee's father. Her then fiancé Jesse Grund took on the mantle for Caylee's father for a while. It was found that Grund was not the father after a DNA test. Anthony later left with Caylee, after a confrontation with her mother. She then moved into her boyfriend's house (Miller, 2020).

Criminal Behavior

In July 2008, Caylee was reported missing by her grandmother, Cindy Anthony. Casey Anthony had told her boyfriend that she had dropped Caylee with a nanny when she was living with him. It is to be noted that none of her family has met this nanny. Anthony had told her parents that it was easy for her and Caylee to live with the nanny in the nanny's apartment which was near Universal Studios where Anthony worked. She later told her mother that the nanny would bring Caylee to her as she was going on a work trip. Cindy Anthony did not meet her granddaughter for these six days. Anthony later told Cindy that the nanny had met with an accident and that is why both she and Caylee were unable to drop by. Anthony evaded her mother's subsequent requests for meeting or talking with Caylee, making up excuses each time.

On July 19, 2008, Cindy and George Anthony received a letter from a tow station in Orlando where Casey Anthony's car was abandoned. On recovery, the car smelled of decomposing human remains, which prompted Cindy Anthony to report her granddaughter missing. Anthony who was living with her boyfriend at this time was questioned by the police to whom she reported that the nanny had kidnapped her child. She could not provide any information of the nanny and it was later found that even her job at Universal Studios was a lie. Casey Anthony was arrested as a suspect in Caylee's disappearance and was later bailed. She remained pleasant as ever without any worry for her missing daughter. After months of searching Caylee Anthony's remains were found a few miles away from the Anthony house (Moran, 2019).

Casey Anthony, who was initially uncooperative and provided misleading information, was eventually charged with first-degree murder. The prosecution argued that Casey had deliberately killed Caylee, suggesting motives such as avoiding parental responsibilities or personal gain. They presented evidence of Casey's behavior during the investigation, including her partying and lack of concern for her missing daughter, as indicative of guilt (Belich, 2011).

The defense, led by Jose Baez, countered by presenting an alternative theory: that Caylee accidentally drowned in the family pool, and Casey's subsequent behavior was a result of panic and denial. They argued that the prosecution's case was based largely on circumstantial evidence and that there was no concrete proof linking Casey directly to the murder (Belich, 2011). The trial was marked by intense media coverage, public outrage, and a polarizing debate over the evidence presented.

Psychological Profile

Casey Anthony grew up in Orlando, Florida, in a family that seemed stable on the surface but reportedly dealt with complex internal dynamics. Her father, George Anthony, a former police officer, and her mother, Cindy Anthony, a registered nurse, projected an image of a close-knit family. However, reports and testimonies later revealed an environment rife with control issues, boundary challenges, and emotional manipulation. Her parents, especially Cindy, were described as overbearing, and there was a possible element of dysfunction that may have hindered Casey's emotional development (Moran, 2019).

Psychologically, growing up in a controlling environment can often contribute to a sense of rebellion and deceit as coping mechanisms. Casey's behavior as a teenager reportedly included frequent lying and manipulative tactics, suggesting early signs of detachment from accountability and an inclination to create alternative realities as a way to navigate difficult situations (Moran, 2019). Some psychological theories propose that such dynamics in adolescence can lead to personality traits associated with deception and a disregard for societal norms.

One of the most notable aspects of Casey Anthony's profile is her consistent pattern of lying and manipulation, both before and after Caylee's disappearance. Casey exhibited a tendency to lie about significant aspects of her life, often fabricating intricate stories. For example, she repeatedly lied about her employment, insisting that she worked at Universal Studios even when this was proven false, and invented elaborate details about friends and babysitters who did not exist (Moran, 2019).

Psychologically, habitual lying and fabrication may suggest traits associated with narcissistic and histrionic personality disorders, where individuals display a disregard for truth in favor of self-serving narratives. In such cases, lies are often used as a defense mechanism to maintain control over others' perceptions, avoid responsibility, or seek validation. Casey's lies extended beyond self-preservation; they seemed to construct an elaborate personal narrative that fed her need for attention and sympathy, traits often found in narcissistic or histrionic personality types.

Another aspect central to Casey's psychological profile is her apparent emotional detachment and lack of remorse following her daughter's disappearance. During the 31 days Caylee was missing, Casey failed to report her absence to authorities and instead continued with her daily life, engaging in social activities, attending parties, and even getting a tattoo reading "Bella Vita," meaning "Beautiful Life" (Moran, 2019). Her detachment and seemingly carefree demeanor raised serious questions about her emotional and psychological state.

This behavior suggests a profound level of emotional disconnect and possibly psychopathic traits, characterized by a lack of empathy, guilt, or remorse. Individuals with psychopathic tendencies are often unable to form meaningful emotional attachments, even with close family members, and tend to view relationships primarily in terms of their utility rather than genuine connection. In Casey's case, this emotional detachment could point to an inability or unwillingness to feel the expected emotional responses to her daughter's death, aligning her behavior with traits often found in psychopathy or sociopathy.

Some theorists have argued that Casey's emotional response—or lack thereof—could also point to a form of dissociation, a psychological mechanism where individuals detach from reality to cope with traumatic events. However, dissociation alone typically doesn't account for the ongoing patterns of lying, manipulation, and deception evident in her profile.

Casey Anthony's behavior reflects several narcissistic traits, including a sense of entitlement, a need for admiration, and an unwillingness to accept responsibility. Narcissistic personality disorder (NPD) is characterized by an inflated sense of self-importance, a lack of empathy, and a strong need for validation, often leading individuals to prioritize their desires above those of others. Casey's decision to continue her social life and seek personal satisfaction during her daughter's absence rather than focusing on finding her suggests a grandiose self-perception and inability to consider others' needs.

Her need for attention was highlighted in her trial, where she reportedly appeared to enjoy the media attention and public spectacle surrounding her case. This behavior aligns with narcissistic traits, as individuals with NPD often enjoy being the center of attention, even in negative contexts. In this sense, Casey may have derived a sense of self-worth from the public scrutiny, regardless of its implications for her reputation or the impact on her family.

Family testimonies suggested a codependent relationship between Casey and her mother, Cindy, which may have fueled Casey's behavior. Cindy reportedly played a controlling role in Casey's life, often managing aspects of her day-to-day activities, including caregiving for Caylee. This dynamic may have created a sense of dependency in Casey, who perhaps resented the lack of control over her life but also relied heavily on Cindy's support.

In cases of codependency, individuals can struggle with feelings of inadequacy and powerlessness, leading to resentment and passive-aggressive behavior. Casey may have exhibited these traits by rebelling in covert ways, such as lying and creating alternative realities, as a means of exerting control. Furthermore, a dependent personality may struggle with a deep need for approval, which could partially explain her behavior, as she sought validation from social circles and even the media during her trial.

While no official diagnosis has been given, some observers have speculated that Casey Anthony may exhibit traits associated with borderline personality disorder (BPD), a complex condition marked by intense emotional instability, fear of abandonment, impulsivity, and unstable relationships. One of the core features of BPD is a pervasive fear of abandonment, which can lead individuals to take extreme measures to avoid real or perceived rejection. In Casey Anthony's case, the dynamics within her family—particularly her relationship with her parents, George and Cindy Anthony—were complicated and fraught with tension. Cindy was reportedly controlling, and some speculate that Casey may have felt stifled or judged, especially as a young single mother living in her parents' home.

If Casey did experience intense abandonment fears, these may have exacerbated her tendency to lie and manipulate to maintain control and protect her self-image. Her unstable relationship with her family, particularly with her mother, might also reflect the tumultuous interpersonal patterns typical of BPD, where individuals alternate between idealization and devaluation in relationships, unable to maintain a stable or consistent view of others.

Possible Treatment

Addressing Casey Anthony's psychological issues would involve a multifaceted approach. Cognitive-behavioral therapy (CBT) could be beneficial in managing her manipulative tendencies and emotional instability. Therapy would aim to help her develop healthier coping mechanisms and address underlying personality disorders. However, the deeply entrenched nature of personality disorders presents significant challenges, and traditional therapeutic approaches may have limited effectiveness (Hickey, 2016).

Additionally, long-term psychotherapy and possibly pharmacological interventions might be necessary to address symptoms of anxiety and emotional dysregulation. The effectiveness of such treatments would depend on Casey's willingness to engage in the therapeutic process and her capacity for self-reflection and change (Hickey, 2016).

Captivation and Trial

The Casey Anthony trial began in May 2011 and quickly became one of the most widely followed trials in US history. The trial featured a dramatic presentation of evidence, including forensic testimony and psychological evaluations. The prosecution's case was built on circumstantial evidence and the portrayal of Casey's behavior as indicative of guilt. The defense focused on creating reasonable doubt by challenging the evidence and presenting an alternative theory of accidental death (Belich, 2011).

In a highly controversial verdict, Casey Anthony was acquitted of the most serious charges, including first-degree murder, but was convicted of four counts of providing false information to law enforcement. The acquittal sparked widespread debate about the legal system's handling of evidence and the impact of media coverage on the trial's outcome (Baden & Homicz, 2012).

Conclusion

The Casey Anthony trial serves as a complex case study in forensic psychology, illustrating the challenges of understanding psychological profiles in high-profile legal cases. The case underscores the importance of thorough psychological evaluations and the impact of media and public opinion on legal proceedings. Understanding Anthony's psychological makeup and the factors influencing the trial's outcome provides valuable insights into the intersection of mental health and criminal justice.

References

Baden, J., & Homicz, L. (2012). *Casey Anthony: Acquittal and aftermath*. Skyhorse Publishing.

Belich, B. (2011). *Inside the Casey Anthony trial*. BenBella Books.

Hickey, E. W. (2016). *Serial murderers and their victims* (7th ed.). Cengage Learning.

Miller, A. (2020). *Casey Anthony: Mother of disappeared Caylee Anthony*. Tiffany Hughes.

Perry, M. (2009). *The Casey Anthony case: A comprehensive review*. Random House.

PART V

Notable Cases and Controversies

17

THE BURARI DEATHS

Introduction

The Burari deaths, a haunting incident from Delhi in 2018, involved the deaths of 11 members of the Chundawat family under mysterious and tragic circumstances. This case explores the intricate blend of psychological, cultural, and familial factors that contributed to the events, offering profound insights into how mental health and societal influences can converge in extreme outcomes.

Background

In July 2018, the Chundawat family was found dead in their home in Burari, Delhi. The victims—comprising three generations—were discovered hanging in a manner that initially suggested a mass suicide. The family, known for their religious devotion and close-knit dynamics, had a history of communal rituals and strong belief systems that were pivotal in the investigation (Bansal, 2018).

Reports indicated that the family had been involved in a series of religious rituals, which included daily prayers and religious gatherings. Their socio-economic status was modest, and they were perceived as a well-integrated part of their local community. The investigation revealed that the family had been planning for the "afterlife," and this context played a crucial role in understanding the events leading to their deaths (Bansal, 2018).

The Chundawat family migrated from Tohana in Haryana to Sant Nagar, Burari, in the 1990s. They had a grocery store which expanded to two as years passed. The head of the family was Bhopal Singh and his wife was Narayni

DOI: 10.4324/9781003602927-22

Devi. They had three children, Bhuvanesh, Pratibha, and Lalit. As time went on Bhuvanesh married Savita and had two daughters, Nitu and Monu, and a son, Dhruv. Lalit got married to Tina and had a son, Shivam. Pratibha got married and widowed. She had a daughter Priyanka. The neighbors describe the family as close-knit and religious (Meghana & Tanush, 2023).

In the year 2007, Bhopal Singh, who was the pillar of the family, passed away. This was a huge blow to the entire family and more specifically to Lalit. Lalit had lost his voice in an accident and his father's death made him more introverted. On a prayer organized as part of the death ritual for Bhopal Singh, Lalit regained his voice and started chanting Om. Lalit later claimed that his father came to him in his sleep and gave him instructions as to how the family should behave and gave guidance on major decisions of the family. He used to have episodes of possession, where his actions and voice would become similar to Bhopal Singh (G & B A, 2023).

In the following years Lalit took on the position of the family head, leading the family to prosperity. He continued to receive instructions from his late father through his dreams. He made detailed notes of these instructions in diaries (written by Priyanka and Nitu on Lalit's instructions) that later provided great insight into his delusions. The whole family, regardless of young and old, believed in Lalit's words and followed his rules on how to conduct themselves. The experts who conducted the psychological autopsy of the family suggested the idea of shared psychosis by the family. This possible shared psychosis escalated to the collective suicide by the family days before the marriage of the eldest granddaughter, Priyanka (G & B A, 2023).

Criminal Behavior

The circumstances of the deaths involved all 11 family members being found hanging, with some in the seated position, which suggested a ritualistic element. Handwritten notes found in the home hinted at a belief in divine intervention, and the family's actions were initially interpreted as a collective psychotic episode or a religious delusion. The case was initially treated as a mass suicide, with investigations pointing toward a shared delusion among the family members (Bansal, 2018; Sharma, 2018).

The meticulous nature of the deaths, including the arrangement of the bodies and the presence of religious texts, suggested that the family might have been influenced by a collective psychosis. This phenomenon, where a group shares a delusional belief system, played a significant role in shaping the understanding of the case (Sharma, 2018).

The ten members of the Chundawat family were found hanging in their courtyard by neighbors on July 1, 2019. The only living member in the house was the pet dog that was tied up on the terrace. All the family members had duct tape on their mouths and cotton balls in their ears and they were all blindfolded. Each of their hands was bound with telephone wires and both hands and feet were bound for the children. The eldest member of the family, Narayani Devi, was found in another room with strangulation marks around her neck. The only person who seemed to have shown some form of struggle was Bhuvanesh. Later investigations into Lalit's diaries found that the family was doing a ritual called "badh tapasya." The family expected to survive the hangings and please the Gods with this ritual (G & B A, 2023).

Psychological Profile

The Burari deaths, involving the mysterious demise of 11 members of the Chundawat family in New Delhi, India, in 2018, have captivated psychological, criminological, and sociocultural analyses due to the eerie circumstances surrounding the case. This complex tragedy involved the deaths of three generations of a single family, discovered hanging in their home under conditions that many interpreted as ritualistic or delusional. The unusual case raised questions about collective psychosis, delusional belief systems, and the profound impacts of family dynamics and trauma.

The Chundawat family consisted of 11 members spanning three generations, living together in a modest home in Burari, Delhi. In July 2018, the bodies were discovered in their residence, with ten family members hanging in a manner that suggested a ritualistic or planned act. The 11th family member, the 77-year-old matriarch, was found in another room, lying on the floor. The case stunned the public due to its chilling elements, including handwritten notes found in the home detailing what seemed to be instructions or rules related to the family's "ritual." These notes, allegedly written by Lalit Chundawat, the youngest son, contained instructions for the entire family to perform specific acts, purportedly for "salvation" or "prosperity." Lalit, a central figure in the case, was thought to be highly influential in leading the family toward this disturbing end (Bansal, 2018).

From a psychological perspective, Lalit's influence over the family plays a crucial role in understanding the Burari deaths. After the death of his father, Lalit reportedly began experiencing traumatic symptoms and psychotic episodes, including auditory hallucinations in which he believed his deceased father was speaking to him. In time, these hallucinatory experiences grew into delusions where he saw himself as a medium for his father's spirit. Lalit reportedly interpreted his hallucinations as spiritual directives meant to guide the family's well-being and security (Bansal, 2018).

These hallucinatory experiences and the resulting delusions align with the features of a psychotic disorder, such as schizophrenia, or a delusional disorder characterized by themes of control and religious or spiritual significance. Lalit's perception that his father's spirit was communicating with him might have originated from unresolved grief and a deep-seated need for control in the wake of his father's death. His belief that he had to carry out his father's "commands" for the family's benefit became an obsessive, life-encompassing conviction, one that he eventually shared with the entire family.

Lalit's influence over the family and their willingness to adhere to his instructions suggest an environment marked by dependency, loyalty, and perhaps a tendency toward conformity. Indian culture, particularly within close-knit families, often emphasizes obedience and respect for elders. This cultural context may have played a role in why the family followed Lalit's directives unquestioningly. The family likely viewed these actions as necessary for achieving harmony or protecting themselves from perceived dangers.

In addition to Lalit's influence, there is evidence that the family may have developed a form of *shared psychotic disorder* or *folie à plusieurs*—a rare psychiatric syndrome where one person's delusion becomes shared among close associates (G & B A, 2023). This condition is facilitated by prolonged social isolation, intense family bonds, and authoritarian control within a group. In the Burari case, Lalit's psychotic beliefs about communicating with his father seemed to spread through the family, forming a collective narrative in which their actions, no matter how extreme, were justified as part of a spiritual mission.

A shared psychotic disorder thrives in a context where an influential individual—often with psychotic symptoms—can impose their beliefs on impressionable or dependent individuals. Within the Chundawat family, Lalit's charismatic authority and the respect he commanded allowed his beliefs to integrate deeply into the family's shared psyche. This environment, combined with the family's possible social isolation, could have intensified their dependence on each other and contributed to their acceptance of Lalit's delusional beliefs.

The Burari case also highlights the intersection of mental health, superstition, and traditional values in Indian society. Beliefs in spirits, ancestral intervention, and rituals for spiritual protection are still pervasive across many Indian communities. Lalit's belief that his deceased father was guiding him may have resonated with culturally ingrained beliefs about spirituality and the afterlife, reducing the likelihood of skepticism within the family. The family's compliance could have been reinforced by their faith in Lalit's guidance as a medium and the idea that these rituals were integral to their survival and prosperity.

Furthermore, mental health remains stigmatized in many parts of India, leading to reluctance among families to seek psychiatric help. If the Chundawat family had sought mental health treatment for Lalit, it is possible that his psychotic symptoms could have been managed, preventing the tragic events. However, it is likely that their awareness of mental health services was limited, or they felt apprehensive about seeking help due to the stigma associated with mental illness.

The rituals detailed in the notes discovered at the scene suggest a need for structure, control, and obedience within the family. Each instruction specified certain steps for each member, reflecting how Lalit's influence over the family had manifested in a system of rules that symbolized unity and faith in his "vision." These instructions were carried out with meticulous care, indicating a level of devotion and perhaps a psychological mechanism where adherence to these rituals provided the family with comfort or stability in their faith.

The nature of these rituals also aligns with compulsive or obsessive behaviors often seen in religious or spiritual delusions. Lalit's need to repeat and enforce specific actions points to obsessive tendencies where performing rituals would reinforce his delusions and alleviate anxiety. This belief system became a shared framework within which the family's collective fears and anxieties were managed, however maladaptively.

Lalit's mental health decline, which seemingly began after his father's death, underlines the psychological impact of trauma and unresolved grief. Losing a significant figure can destabilize individuals who are psychologically vulnerable, as seen in Lalit's case. His trauma response took the form of auditory hallucinations, which, left untreated, evolved into delusional beliefs. The lack of emotional or psychological support for Lalit, coupled with his inability to process his grief healthily, turned his delusions into a family tragedy.

The Burari deaths serve as a stark reminder of the importance of mental health awareness, especially in societies where mental illness is stigmatized. The case illustrates how untreated psychosis, coupled with cultural factors and familial loyalty, can create tragic outcomes. Understanding and addressing mental health symptoms, even when embedded in culturally significant beliefs, is essential to preventing similar cases. It underscores the need for accessible mental health services, education to reduce stigma, and early intervention, particularly for families experiencing signs of shared delusional disorders or other forms of collective psychological distress.

Possible Treatment

Addressing cases involving shared psychosis and collective delusions requires a multifaceted approach. Preventive measures should include community mental health initiatives and increased awareness of the impact of cultural practices on psychological well-being. Effective treatment would involve both individual and group therapy, focusing on breaking down delusional beliefs and fostering healthier coping mechanisms (Srinivasan, 2019).

Community support systems and mental health education are crucial in preventing similar tragedies. Efforts should be directed toward improving mental health literacy and creating support networks that can intervene early when signs of collective psychosis or severe psychological distress are evident (Kumar & Sharma, 2020).

Captivation and Trial

The Burari case garnered extensive media attention due to its disturbing nature and the complexity of the investigation. The case revealed the interplay between cultural beliefs and psychological factors, and the media coverage highlighted the need for a nuanced understanding of such phenomena. Investigators faced challenges in deciphering the motivations behind the deaths and understanding the family's beliefs and practices (Bansal, 2018; Kumar & Sharma, 2020).

The police ruled out homicide quickly as evidence in the form of Lalit's diary and CCTV footage were recovered. Lalit's diary had detailed descriptions of how each family member would hang themselves for the ritual in the shape of a Banyan tree. Even the description of Narayani Devi joining the ritual in the next room was consistent with how her body was recovered. CCTV footage of July 28, 2019, shows Lalit's wife and son buying four stools. Another footage of Tina and Nitu buying the rest of the equipment used for hanging was also recovered on July 30. The psychological autopsy concluded that this was neither a suicide nor a homicide but a tragic culmination of a shared psychotic disorder (G & B A, 2023).

Conclusion

The Burari tragedy underscores the profound impact of cultural and psychological factors on extreme outcomes. It serves as a critical reminder of the need for comprehensive mental health education and community support to address and prevent such complex cases. Understanding the interplay between mental health, cultural practices, and familial dynamics is essential for developing effective strategies to mitigate similar risks in the future.

References

Bansal, A. (2018). *The Burari deaths: Unraveling the mystery*. HarperCollins.

Kumar, S., & Sharma, R. (2020). *Mental health and cultural influences: Lessons from the Burari case*. Sage Publications.

Meghana, G., & Tanush, B. A. (2023). From belief to tragedy: Unveiling the layers of the Burari case. *Jus Corpus Law Journal*, *4*(1). https://doi-ds.org/doilink/10.2023-86198134/juscorpuslawjournal/v4/i1/6779

Sharma, V. (2018). *The Burari deaths: A forensic and psychological analysis*. Routledge.

Srinivasan, V. (2019). *Mental health and cultural influences: Lessons from the Burari case*. Oxford University Press.

18

THE CASE OF WEST MEMPHIS THREE

Introduction

The West Memphis Three case is a profound illustration of potential miscarriages of justice within the American legal system. This case study delves into the psychological profiles of Damien Echols, Jason Baldwin, and Jessie Misskelley, exploring their backgrounds, criminal behavior, and the factors that led to their controversial and wrongful convictions.

Background

In 1993, three 8-year-old boys—Stevie Branch, Christopher Byers, and Michael Moore—were found murdered in West Memphis, Arkansas. The case quickly garnered national attention, partly due to the sensationalized notion of Satanic ritualistic murder. Teenagers Damien Echols, Jason Baldwin, and Jessie Misskelley were arrested and charged with the murders, largely due to their nonconformist behavior and Echols' known interest in the occult (Leveritt, 2002; Bogira, 2009).

Echols, in particular, was an outsider who dressed differently and was interested in occult practices, which fueled public and media speculation about his involvement in the murders. The case against them was heavily influenced by this moral panic despite the absence of substantive evidence linking them to the crime (Leveritt, 2002).

Michael Wayne Hutchison aka Damien Echols, was born on December 11, 1974. His parents divorced when he was 8 and he moved around with his mother till they settled in West Memphis with his stepfather. He grew up in poverty and had been displaced a lot as a child. He was a misfit among his

DOI: 10.4324/9781003602927-23

peers. He wore black clothes all year round and identified himself as a Wicca member. He wrote dark love poems and gave himself the name Damien to fit in with the witchcraft community (Leveritt, 2002).

Charles Jason Baldwin, who goes by his middle name, also had a troubled childhood. His father left when he was a child, and he lived with his mother and stepfather. He was more artistically inclined and could have done better with his study. As a teenager, he wore black T-shirts and listened to metallica. Baldwin befriended Echols, and the two had burglary records in their files. Jessi Miskelley Jr., the last member of the West Memphis Three, was also a misfit with a bad temper. Not much is known about his home life as a child or teenager (Leveritt, 2002).

Criminal Behavior

The prosecution's case was primarily based on coerced confessions, dubious forensic evidence, and the defendants' unconventional lifestyles. Jessie Misskelley, who had an IQ of 72 and was easily coerced, provided a confession after hours of intense interrogation. This confession was riddled with inconsistencies and later deemed unreliable. There was no physical evidence connecting the defendants to the crime scene, yet they were convicted largely due to the confessions and the moral panic surrounding the case (Bogira, 2009; Hickey, 2016).

The case exemplifies how psychological pressure and the criminal justice system's flaws can lead to wrongful convictions. The convictions of the West Memphis Three were heavily criticized for relying on questionable methods and ignoring exculpatory evidence (Hickey, 2016).

Three elementary school students, Steve Branch, Michael Moore, and Christopher Byers, went missing from their neighborhood in West Memphis. They were last seen around 6:30 pm by the neighbors and were reported missing around 7:00 pm the same day. The police and community began searching for them around 8:00 pm around the Robin Hood Hills where they were last seen. It was not until the next noon that the police found the remains of the three boys in a drainage ditch near the Robin Hood Hills. All three boys were naked and their hands and feet were bound behind their backs with their shoe laces. Most of their clothing was discovered near the body disposal site. Autopsies of the body revealed that two of the boys died of drowning and multiple injuries and Byers died of multiple injuries. There were initial suspicions of rape because of the semen sample found in the pants of one of the boys, but no evidence of it was found in autopsy. The injuries on the boys and castration of one of the victims, Byers, was reported to be made with a knife wound by prosecution expert witnesses (Leveritt, 2002).

Psychological Profile

The West Memphis Three—Damien Echols, Jason Baldwin, and Jessie Misskelley—were teenagers when they were accused and convicted of the 1993 murders of three young boys in West Memphis, Arkansas (Leveritt, 2002). Their case became infamous not only due to the brutality of the crime but also due to the accusations of Satanic ritual abuse that dominated their trials, leading to a highly controversial investigation and convictions based largely on circumstantial evidence and confessions under duress. Psychological profiles of each of these young men highlight their unique vulnerabilities and the various factors that contributed to their wrongful convictions, as well as their psychological resilience throughout their incarceration.

Damien Echols, the most visible and vocal of the three, was regarded as an "outsider" in his community. He was known for his alternative style, interest in heavy metal music, and exploration of occult topics—interests that marked him as different in a conservative and religious town like West Memphis. Echols' psychological profile reveals a young man who sought identity and self-expression through rebellion against societal norms, leading to misunderstandings and prejudices that fueled suspicions against him.

At 18, Echols displayed characteristics often associated with adolescent countercultural rebellion. He dressed in black, wrote dark poetry, and spoke openly about his interest in Wicca and pagan practices. These traits became the focus of the prosecution's case against him, painting him as a "devil-worshiper" in an environment steeped in moral panic over Satanic ritual abuse. His nonconformity and unconventional beliefs contributed to his community's mistrust and reinforced his feeling of alienation.

Psychological assessments of Echols indicate that he exhibited high levels of resilience, intelligence, and self-awareness. Despite the intense scrutiny and mistreatment he faced, Echols remained intellectually curious and developed a strong sense of self. His writings from prison show a deep philosophical and introspective quality, suggesting that he coped with his isolation by finding meaning and purpose through intellectual exploration. Over time, he turned to meditation and spiritual practices, which provided psychological support and helped him endure the hardships of death row.

Echols' profile suggests an individual who, although misunderstood and scapegoated, possessed the mental fortitude to withstand an extraordinary ordeal. His eventual release was partially due to his willingness to communicate his experiences to the outside world and raise awareness of his wrongful conviction, demonstrating both resilience and a desire for justice.

Jason Baldwin, the youngest of the three, was just 16 at the time of his arrest. In contrast to Echols, Baldwin's personality was more reserved, and he displayed few signs of rebellion or resistance against societal norms. He was a good student with aspirations of becoming an architect and was considered by friends and family as respectful, quiet, and hard-working. His psychological profile reflects a young man who, though introverted and somewhat impressionable, was grounded in traditional aspirations.

Baldwin's personality made him particularly vulnerable in the context of the investigation. Lacking a strong, assertive personality, he was likely more easily manipulated and found himself implicated largely due to his association with Echols, his best friend. His passive nature and loyalty to his friends made him an unlikely candidate to resist or actively challenge the authorities, rendering him susceptible to the flawed narrative that law enforcement built around his character and friendships.

During his time in prison, Baldwin exhibited characteristics associated with high psychological resilience, patience, and adaptability. He worked to educate himself and maintained hope, eventually choosing not to adopt the "Alford plea" initially because he did not want to falsely admit guilt, even though doing so would have secured his release sooner. This demonstrated strong moral principles and a sense of integrity, rare qualities for someone who spent much of his formative years incarcerated. In his profile, Baldwin's psychological strength emerges not through rebellion or assertiveness, but through his quiet endurance and loyalty. His reserved nature and aversion to conflict likely made him appear more compliant, but his intellectual curiosity and integrity helped him endure his sentence with dignity and a sense of hope for eventual exoneration.

Jessie Misskelley, Jr., the third member of the West Memphis Three, presents the most complex psychological profile due to his intellectual and emotional vulnerabilities. At 17, Misskelley had an IQ of around 72, placing him in the borderline intellectual functioning range, which made him highly susceptible to suggestion, manipulation, and influence from authority figures. This vulnerability played a central role in the legal case against him, as he provided a coerced confession under hours of police interrogation without a lawyer or parent present. His limited cognitive functioning, combined with his desire to please authority figures, rendered him highly vulnerable to leading questions and suggestive tactics employed by law enforcement.

Misskelley's psychological profile reflects traits often seen in individuals with intellectual disabilities, including heightened suggestibility, eagerness to please, and an impaired ability to comprehend the full implications of his actions. During his interrogation, Misskelley repeatedly changed his story, indicating confusion and a lack of understanding of the gravity of the situation. His confession was filled with inconsistencies, and much of it was prompted by leading questions, suggesting that he was coerced into saying what he thought the police wanted to hear.

Despite these challenges, Misskelley displayed significant emotional strength in enduring his sentence. His mental limitations, however, complicated his ability to adapt to the harsh conditions of prison life. His time in incarceration was marked by moments of confusion and struggle, particularly as he had difficulty understanding the legal complexities of his case. Nevertheless, Misskelley managed to maintain a connection with his family and friends and relied on their support to cope with his isolation and the challenges of prison. Misskelley's profile suggests a highly vulnerable individual whose limited intellectual capacity made him easy prey for those looking to assign blame quickly. His psychological resilience was weaker compared to Echols and Baldwin, but his reliance on his social support network allowed him to endure and find stability amidst his profound struggles.

The West Memphis Three, as a group, demonstrate how varied psychological profiles can contribute to resilience in the face of extreme adversity. Despite their differences, each young man found ways to cope, adapt, and ultimately survive. Echols' intellectual pursuits and spiritual exploration, Baldwin's quiet determination and integrity, and Misskelley's reliance on his support system reveal different pathways to resilience and psychological survival. Their collective bond and shared experiences of hardship helped them endure nearly two decades of wrongful incarceration. Their eventual release and exoneration underscore the critical importance of understanding how vulnerabilities, psychological profiles, and social biases can lead to wrongful convictions. Each young man's psychological profile reveals how their unique characteristics were used against them in the legal system, resulting in the tragic miscarriage of justice that took years to correct.

The West Memphis Three case serves as a powerful example of resilience in the face of systemic failure and the ways in which psychological resilience can be fostered, even in the most adverse conditions. Through their unique profiles, we gain insight into how vulnerable individuals can adapt and survive under extreme circumstances, relying on personal strengths, external support, and, ultimately, the pursuit of justice.

Possible Treatment

Effective treatment for the West Memphis Three would have needed to address both their individual psychological needs and the broader systemic issues affecting their case. Damien Echols could have benefited from cognitive-behavioral therapy (CBT) to address antisocial traits and emotional distress. Jessie Misskelley required specialized support for his intellectual disabilities and protection from coercive interrogation techniques. For Baldwin, a focus on trauma-informed care might have been beneficial (Hickey, 2016).

Addressing systemic issues in criminal justice, such as wrongful convictions and coercion, requires comprehensive reforms, including better interrogation practices, improved forensic methods, and enhanced legal representation for vulnerable individuals (Dempsey, 2012).

Captivation and Trial

The West Memphis Three's trial was marked by sensationalist media coverage and legal irregularities. The public's fixation on the idea of Satanic rituals played a significant role in shaping the prosecution's case and the jury's perception. In 2011, after new evidence emerged, the three were released from prison under an Alford plea. This plea allowed them to maintain their innocence while acknowledging that the prosecution had sufficient evidence to convict them. The case continues to be a stark example of wrongful conviction and the influence of public hysteria on legal outcomes (Leveritt, 2002; Bogira, 2009).

The police during their initial investigation focused on Echols, Baldwin, and Misskelley. They reasoned that there was a Satanic component to the murders and the three teens fit as suspects to this narration. Echols and Baldwin were close friends and Echols had ties to the Wicca. Misskelley, on the other hand, was aggressive as a teenager and was involved in fights at school. All three were questioned by the police and an allegedly coerced confession was elicited from Misskelley. This led to the arrest of the three teens even though no physical evidence tied them to the murders. The prosecution also had a witness Vicky Hutcheston who gave a statement that her son who was the playmate of the three victims had seen satanists killing them in a playhouse. The defense tried to argue that Misskelley's confession was coerced and the knowledge of the crime scene that incriminated the other two was only limited to public knowledge of the case. The verdict of the trial was that Echols was sentenced to death, Misskelley to life imprisonment plus 20 years, and Baldwin to life imprisonment. In the following years new evidence including DNA evidence, foreman and jury misconduct, and nonmatching tooth imprints came into the picture that would ultimately lead to the exoneration of the three suspects (Leveritt, 2002).

Conclusion

The West Memphis Three case underscores the critical importance of fair legal processes and the profound impact of social prejudices on justice. By understanding their psychological profiles and the factors leading to their wrongful convictions, we gain valuable insights into the need for reforms in the criminal justice system to prevent such miscarriages of justice in the future.

References

Bogira, S. (2009). *A vengeance in the heartland: The West Memphis Three case*. University of Chicago Press.

Dempsey, J. S. (2012). *The justice game: Lessons from wrongful convictions*. Oxford University Press.

Hickey, E. W. (2016). *Serial murderers and their victims* (7th ed.). Cengage Learning.

Leveritt, M. (2002). *Devil's knot: The true story of the West Memphis Three*. Atria Books.

19
JONBENÉT RAMSEY CASE

Introduction

The JonBenét Ramsey case remains one of the most perplexing unsolved mysteries in modern criminal history. This case study delves into the psychological profiles of the key figures involved, examining their backgrounds, criminal behaviors, and the myriad factors contributing to the case's enduring enigma.

Background

JonBenét Patricia Ramsey, a 6-year-old beauty pageant contestant, was found dead in her Boulder, Colorado, home on December 26, 1996. Her murder shocked the nation and captivated media attention due to her family's high profile and the puzzling circumstances of her death. JonBenét was discovered with a garrote around her neck and signs of blunt force trauma, along with a ransom note found at the scene. Despite extensive investigations, the case remains unsolved, and no conclusive evidence has definitively linked any family member to the crime (Ramsey & Ramsey, 2000; Thomas, 2009).

The Ramsey family, including JonBenét's parents, Patsy and John Ramsey, became the primary focus of the investigation due to inconsistencies in their statements and behavior. The investigation was further complicated by the intense media scrutiny and public speculation surrounding the case (Baker, 2009).

Patsy Ramsey participated in multiple beauty pageants as a child and won the title of Miss Virginia as a young woman. She graduated with a degree in journalism from University of West Virginia. She married John Ramsey, the president of a software company, and had two children with him, Burke

DOI: 10.4324/9781003602927-24

and JonBenét Ramsey. She was a homemaker and was involved with the local churches. The Ramsey family encountered one tragedy after another from 1992 to 1993, when John Ramsey's daughter from a previous family passed away in a car accident and Patsy Ramsey was subsequently diagnosed with ovarian cancer. Patsy Ramsey, post her recovery from cancer in 1995, enrolled her daughter in child beauty pageant competitions and JonBenét Ramsey managed to win a series of pageant titles. JonBenét Ramsey was 6 years old at the time of her kidnapping and was attending kindergarten.

Criminal Behavior

JonBenét's murder involved a complex crime scene with a garrote used to strangle her and blunt force trauma indicating a violent struggle. The ransom note left at the scene suggested a botched kidnapping, but the lack of physical evidence linking the family to the crime created a cloud of suspicion and confusion (Thomas, 2009; Kolar, 2012).

The investigation initially centered on the Ramsey family due to behavioral inconsistencies and the discovery of the ransom note, but as time progressed, the focus shifted to other theories, including the possibility of an intruder. Despite numerous suspects and theories, the case remains unresolved (Kolar, 2012).

JonBenét Ramsey was reported missing by Patsy Ramsey in the morning of December 26, 1996. She reported having found an uncharacteristically lengthy (two and half page long) ransom note demanding $180,000 for the return of JonBenét Ramsey. A neighbor had later reported that he had seen the kitchen of Ramsey house lit and another neighbor had heard a scream of a young girl around the same time. The police found no sign of forced entry to the Ramsey household and John Ramsey was instructed to arrange the money for the ransom. The police never conducted further searches of the house. It was about 1 pm when John Ramsey and his friend were asked by the police to check if anything was missing from the house. It is then that John Ramsey found the remains of his daughter in the basement. Her hands and neck were wrapped by nylon wire, her mouth was duct taped, and she was covered with a white blanket. John Ramsey carried his daughter upstairs, which led to the contamination of the crime scene. Autopsy found that JonBenét Ramsey died due to asphyxiation and head injury. There were signs of sexual assault though no semen sample were recovered (Thomas & Davis, 2011).

Psychological Profile

John Ramsey, JonBenét's father, exhibited a markedly different reaction to his daughter's death, characterized by a controlled and composed exterior. In situations of intense trauma, this coping style is often seen as a form of "emotional suppression," where individuals maintain a calm and stoic demeanor in order to manage their inner turmoil. However, this does not indicate a lack of grief or emotional response; rather, it reflects a psychological mechanism to protect oneself from being overwhelmed by emotions.

The financial success and social standing of the Ramsey family may have further shaped John's response, as he likely felt an obligation to protect his family's image. For individuals accustomed to control, wealth, and stability, an unexpected and unsolvable tragedy can pose a severe psychological threat, undermining their sense of security. John's reserved response could be interpreted as a form of emotional self-preservation, where he focused on maintaining stability amidst the chaos to prevent further disintegration of his family's lives.

It's also worth noting that John Ramsey was acutely aware of the media's scrutiny, which could have exacerbated his need to appear "strong." The high-profile nature of the case left the Ramsey family exposed to intense public suspicion, effectively putting them on trial in the court of public opinion. John's stoicism may have served as a coping strategy to avoid additional accusations or show vulnerability in a time when the family was under relentless scrutiny.

The trauma experienced by the Ramsey family went beyond individual reactions and influenced the collective family dynamic. The parents were thrust into a highly defensive stance, fighting to protect their family's reputation and innocence. The stress of these accusations and the constant media attention created an environment of "siege mentality," where the family likely felt under attack from both the outside world and law enforcement.

In families dealing with sudden, violent loss, there is often a "psychological splitting" that occurs. This process, observed in traumatic grief, involves compartmentalizing painful memories to prevent emotional collapse. Both John and Patsy likely employed this defense mechanism to keep functioning under the circumstances, although it may have contributed to the perception of them as detached or unfeeling. The media portrayal of the Ramseys as affluent and somewhat removed from ordinary life likely deepened the public's sense of distrust and alienation from the family, reinforcing a narrative that cast them in an unfavorable light.

The public nature of the investigation into JonBenét's death had a profound impact on the Ramsey family's ability to grieve. This situation can be seen as a form of "complicated grief," where the natural grieving process is disrupted by external factors such as suspicion, accusations, and ongoing investigations. The omnipresent media coverage turned the Ramsey family into household names, complicating their psychological ability to process their grief privately. Media scrutiny added an additional layer of stress to an already traumatic situation, intensifying their grief and potentially impacting their mental health.

In addition, the media frenzy surrounding JonBenét's case made it difficult for the family to achieve closure, which is a vital part of the grieving process. Rather than being allowed to mourn privately, the Ramseys became part of a public spectacle that continually revisited their daughter's death, preventing them from putting the traumatic experience behind them. This prolonged exposure to public suspicion is known to exacerbate symptoms of post-traumatic stress and can hinder the healing process.

Burke Ramsey, JonBenét's older brother, was 9 years old at the time of her death. In childhood trauma cases, particularly those involving family members, young individuals often exhibit long-term psychological effects. Burke's young age at the time of the incident likely limited his understanding of the full scope of the events; however, he was still subjected to the aftermath and scrutiny surrounding the case. Over the years, he has shown signs of emotional suppression similar to his father, though his experiences as a child witnessing his family's trauma likely led to psychological effects, such as feelings of isolation, anxiety, and distrust.

The psychological profiles of the Ramsey family underscore the impact of unresolved trauma and public scrutiny. They illustrate how grief and coping mechanisms vary across family members, influenced by personality, cultural expectations, and external pressures. The case highlights how public suspicion and relentless media attention can turn grieving into a form of ongoing psychological siege, with effects that reverberate through each family member.

The Ramseys' experiences also reflect the broader impact of media in high-profile cases, where speculation and sensationalism can disrupt families' attempts to cope with personal tragedies. The case serves as a reminder of the importance of trauma-informed practices in law enforcement and media, emphasizing the need for sensitivity to the unique vulnerabilities of individuals facing public scrutiny in the wake of personal loss.

Possible Treatment

For the Ramsey family, trauma-focused therapy would have been essential in addressing the profound grief and psychological distress resulting from JonBenét's murder. Cognitive-behavioral therapy (CBT) could have helped them manage their emotional responses and develop coping strategies amidst the relentless media attention and investigative pressure. Additionally, support groups for families affected by violent crime could have provided a therapeutic outlet and communal support (Hickey, 2016; Kolar, 2012).

Captivation and Trial

The JonBenét Ramsey case has seen numerous theories and suspects over the years, including potential intruders and familial involvement. Despite extensive investigations and public fascination, no definitive conclusion has been reached. The case continues to captivate both public and professional interest, serving as a poignant reminder of the complexities involved in criminal investigations (Thomas, 2009; Kolar, 2012).

Conclusion

The JonBenét Ramsey case highlights the intricate nature of criminal investigations and the profound impact of media on the pursuit of justice. Analyzing the psychological profiles of the key figures involved offers valuable insights into their behavior and the challenges they faced during the investigation, underscoring the need for thorough and unbiased investigative approaches.

References

Baker, J. (2009). *The case of JonBenét Ramsey: The final chapter*. Macmillan.
Hickey, E. W. (2016). *Serial murderers and their victims* (7th ed.). Cengage Learning.
Kolar, L. (2012). *Foreign faction: Who really Kidnapped JonBenét?* AuthorHouse.
Ramsey, J., & Ramsey, P. (2000). *The death of innocence: JonBenét's parents tell their story*. Thomas Nelson.
Thomas, S. (2009). *JonBenét: Inside the Ramsey murder investigation*. St. Martin's Press.

PART VI

Reflections and Future Directions

20

REFLECTIONS AND INSIGHTS

After examining these compelling case studies, we are left with a tapestry of thoughts and revelations that significantly impact our comprehension of criminal justice systems, human behavior, and the function of forensic psychology in deciphering the complexity of crime.

From the ravenous desire for power and control displayed by serial killers like Jeffrey Dahmer and Ted Bundy to the tragic results of untreated mental illness in cases like Andrea Yates and Aileen Wuornos, we have encountered people motivated by a wide range of reasons throughout our journey. We have seen how familial trauma and social dynamics affect people like the Menendez brothers, whose lives were molded by the atrocities of abuse and neglect.

Significant doubts have been expressed regarding the validity of the evidence, the impact of media sensationalism, and the difficulties involved in jury decision-making in the wake of the trials of O. J. Simpson, Casey Anthony, and the West Memphis Three. We have addressed the confluence of ideology, mental illness, and violence in instances such as the one involving Ted Kaczynski, the Unabomber, whose manifesto exposed the extent of his radicalization and seclusion.

We have learned so much about the minds of both offenders and victims via the lens of forensic psychology, which has helped us understand the complex web of variables that lead to criminal behavior. Forensic psychologists are essential in helping to unravel the complexity of crime and justice, from analyzing personality features and behavioral patterns to looking into societal dynamics and trauma.

These stories serve as a constant reminder of the devastating effects that crime has on people as individuals, as families, and as communities. We have

DOI: 10.4324/9781003602927-26

to work toward a just system that is equitable, fair, and grounded in compassion and understanding. We may strive toward a future where justice is served together with healing and reconciliation for all those impacted by crime by continuing to enhance forensic psychology research and practice.

Ultimately, these case studies provide a moving reminder of the never-ending search for justice, compassion, and the truth in a world full of darkness and hopelessness. By working together, we can create a society in which the rights of the accused are upheld, the voices of the victims are heard, and the scars of the past are healed into hope for a better future.

INDEX

For Product Safety Concerns and Information please contact our EU representative GPSR@taylorandfrancis.com
Taylor & Francis Verlag GmbH, Kaufingerstraße 24, 80331 München, Germany

www.ingramcontent.com/pod-product-compliance
Ingram Content Group UK Ltd.
Pitfield, Milton Keynes, MK11 3LW, UK
UKHW022314250926
475702UK00046B/787
9781032989648